The

DIVERTICULITIS COOKBOOK

28 DAY HELPFUL MEAL PLAN

The Complete Nutrition Guide
to Relieve Diverticular Flare-Ups for a Better Life!

INTRODUCTION OF FODMAP DIET INCLUDED!

ROBERT DICKENS & ANITA ROSE

Table of Contents

Introduction 8

Diverticulitis vs Diverticulosis 9

    When Do I Know I Have Diverticula 9

    The Difference Between Diverticulitis and Diverticulosis 10

        Diverticulosis 10

        Diverticulitis 10

    Am I at Risk? 12

Causes and Symptoms of Diverticulitis 14

    Symptoms of Diverticulitis 14

    How Diverticulitis Is Diagnosed 15

    How Is Diverticulitis Treated? 15

What Is the Role of Food in the Development of Diverticulitis? 16

    Can Nutrition be Used to Manage Diverticulitis? 16

    Stages of Diverticulitis 17

Why Should You Implement a FODMAP Diet? 19

    How Low-FODMAP Diets Work 19

    The 4 FODMAPS Explained 20

    What Foods Can I Eat on a Low-FODMAP Diet? 22

    Who Should Use a Low-FODMAP Diet? 22

    Benefits of a Low-FODMAP Diet 23

    FAQs 25

Diverticula Meal Planning 28

    The Clear Liquid Phase 28

        Components of a Clear Liquid Diet 28

        Clear Liquid Diet Food Plan 29

        The Advantages and Disadvantages of a Clear Liquid Diet 29

        Guidelines for Undergoing a Clear Liquid Diet 30

    The Juicing Diet 30

        How the Juicing Diet Works 31

        Cons of Juicing 31

    The Low-Residue Diet 32

        Meal Plan for Your Low-Fiber Diet 33

        General Guidelines for Following a Low-Residue Diet 33

    Transitional Phase 34

28-Day Meal Plan	36
Creating the Perfect Shopping List	**42**
Acute Phase Foods	42
Recovery Phase Foods	42
Prevention Foods	43
Myths About Diverticular Diseases	**44**
FAQs About Diverticular Diseases	**48**
MEASUREMENT CONVERSIONS	**50**
Recipes	**52**
Clear Fluids	**53**
Breakfast	
Apple Juice — VEGAN	54
Carrot and Apple Juice — VEGAN	55
Green Juice — VEGAN	56
Lunch	
Green Dragon Veggie Juice — VEGAN	59
Tomato Juice — VEGAN	60
Golden Coffee	61
Vegetable Clear Soup — VEGAN	62
Dinner	
Chicken Clear Soup	65
Japanese Clear Soup	66
Sweet Potato Carrot Spiced Juice	67
Vegan Jello — VEGAN	68
Snaks	
Green Smoothie Popsicles — VEGAN	71
Masala Chai Tea — VEGAN	72
Strawberry Soda Syrup — VEGAN	73
Vegan Chai Latte — VEGAN	74
Watermelon Lime Agua Fresca — VEGAN	75
Low-Fiber	**76**
Breakfast	
Almond Meal Blueberry Muffins	77
Greek Yogurt Oatmeal Pancake	78

Lunch

Almond Flour Bread	80
Chicken Fingers	81
Chicken Sour Cream Enchiladas	82
Gluten-free Crustless Pizza	83
Pumpkin Muffin in a Cup	84
Southern Style Cornbread	85
Tomato Pasta `VEGAN`	86
Zucchini Pizza Crust	87

Dinner

BBQ Beef Stir-Fry	89
Cauliflower Rice `VEGAN`	90
Coconut Flour Bread	91
90 Second Bread	92
Spaghetti Sauce With Ground Turkey	93
Sweet Potato Gnocchi `VEGAN`	94

Snaks

Almond and Jam Cookies	97
Almond Cookies `VEGAN`	98
Banana Bread	99
Chocolate Chip Chickpea Blondies `VEGAN`	100
Easy Peanut Butter Cookies	101
Peanut Butter Brownies	102
Peanut Butter Truffle Cookies	103
Oatmeal Peanut Butter Balls `VEGAN`	104
Pumpkin Spice	105
Tiny Peanut Butter Cookies	106

High-Fiber — 108

Breakfast

Apple Pie Oatmeal	109
Banana Buckwheat Pancakes and Compote	110
Black Bean Spinach Quesadilla	111
Chocolate Cherry Egg White Oatmeal	112

Cinnamon French Toast ... 113
Roasted Cranberry Quinoa Oatmeal ... 114
Savory Cheese Oatmeal ... 115

Lunch

Chicken Breast With Kabocha and Kale ... 117
Chicken, Parsnip, and Pomegranate Salad ... 118
Coconut Lentil Soup `VEGAN` 119
Flat-Belly Salad ... 120
Green Curry Tofu Rice `VEGAN` 121
Hearty Vegetable Curry ... 122
Lentil Soup `VEGAN` 123
Marinated Pear and Fennel With Chickpeas ... 124
Spicy Red Lentil Soup `VEGAN` 125
Spiced Tomato Lentil Soup ... 126
Sweet Potato Chili `VEGAN` 127
Sweet Potato Salad ... 128
Swiss Chard Wraps With Chicken ... 129

Dinner

Baked Potato With Ground Beef and Broccoli ... 131
Broccoli Cheddar Brown Rice ... 132
Brussels Sprouts and Sweet Potato Hash ... 133
Flank Steak Tacos ... 134
Greek Chicken Pasta ... 135
Grilled Zucchini Hummus `VEGAN` 136
Parmesan Cauliflower With Chickpeas ... 137
Rainbow Veggie Chili `VEGAN` 138
Roasted Pork Loin With Apple Jus ... 139
Salmon Quinoa and Roasted Brussel Sprouts ... 141
Sheet Pan Salmon ... 142
Spicy Black Bean Burgers ... 143
Superfast Asparagus `VEGAN` 144
Sweet Potato With White Bean Bake `VEGAN` 145
Wilted Kale, Chickpeas, and Quinoa `VEGAN` 146

Snaks

Banana Nuts Overnight Oats	149
Kale and Pear Smoothie	150
Yogurt With Pumpkin Granola	151

Low-FODMAP — 152

Breakfast

Egg Wraps		153
Banana Porridge	VEGAN	154
Banana Oatcakes		155
Pineapple, Strawberry, Raspberry Smoothie	VEGAN	156
Blueberry, Lime, and Coconut Smoothie	VEGAN	157
Crepes and Berries		158

Lunch

Tomato and Green Bean Salad		161
Corn Salad	VEGAN	162
Pesto Noodles		163
Chicken Wrap		164
Quiche in Ham Cups		165
Feta, Chicken, and Pepper Sandwich		166
Rice & Zucchini Slice		167

Dinner

Bolognese		169
Minestrone		170
Vegetable Fried Rice		171
Roasted Pumpkin and Carrot Soup	VEGAN	172
Feta Meatball		173
Spicy Tacos		174
Gnocchi		175
Vegan Curry	VEGAN	176

Snaks

Quinoa Muffins		179
Chocolate Peanut Butter Energy Bites	VEGAN	180
Summer Popsicle	VEGAN	181
Orange Biscuits		182
Coconut Bites		183

| Energy Bars | 184 |

Conclusion **186**

Others books by Robert Dickens **175**

Scan QR code
To Download **10 Extra Recipes**
For Low-Fodmap Diet

Introduction

Diverticulitis is an inflammation of the lining of the digestive system that, sometimes, results in uncomfortable symptoms. Fever, nausea, and constant pain are a few of the symptoms associated with this type of inflammation.

If advised by a doctor, one may rely on the right diet to manage and cure diverticulitis. This dietary approach is merely temporary, as it helps symptoms, such as diarrhea, subside. Nutrition for diverticulitis begins with clear liquids. After some time, the patient must progress to incorporate low-fiber meals into their diet.

This book will explain everything you need to know about diverticulitis—short of needing a professional medical consultation, that is. It will also include a meal plan and shopping list to assist you with your diet.

But you might agree that the most interesting of the chapters in this book are the delicious and easy-to-prepare recipes. They can be made quickly, using affordable ingredients, and will help to relieve and cure the symptoms of diverticulitis.

Chapter 1
Diverticulitis vs Diverticulosis
When Do I Know I Have Diverticula

Diverticula are tiny, bulging pockets that develop around the lining of the digestive system. They usually form around the regions of the lower large intestine, known as the volon. Diverticula is a common condition, especially among those over the age of 40. But they are rarely known to be problematic. Having diverticula means that you suffer from diverticulosis. However, when inflammation occurs in one or several diverticula and, in some cases, infection as well, the condition morphs into diverticulitis. When diverticulitis occurs, you become susceptible to symptoms, such as a substantial change in your typical bowel habits, nausea, fever, and abdominal pain.

Think of diverticula as bubbles or expansions in an area, which are created when the inner tube of a bicycle's tire is filled with more than enough air. The internal pressure in the inner tube is going to rise due to the excessive air pumped in and will result in bubbles or expansions in the weakest areas of the rubber material. In the same vein, any increase in the internal pressure of the colon can lead to bulges or pockets (diverticula) that develop in the weakest areas of the walls of the colon. The sizes of diverticula range from those about the size of peas to expansions that can be measured in centimeters. Although it's possible for diverticula to develop in any region of the colon's inner lining, they tend to be located in the lower left side of the S-shaped segment known as the sigmoid colon.

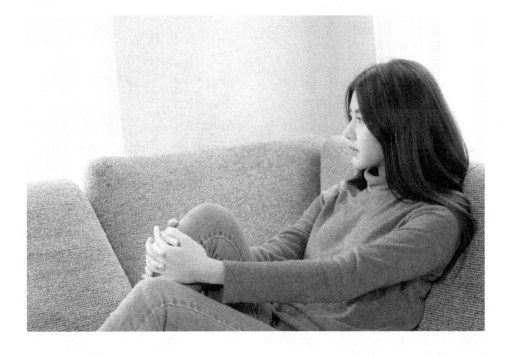

The Difference Between Diverticulitis and Diverticulosis

Diverticulosis

Diverticulosis is the presence of several small pockets or bulges in the colon known as diverticula. These bulges are quite harmless and do not require any form of treatment. Neither do they present symptoms. But, if care is not taken, diverticulosis could spiral into a more dangerous condition. Put simply, if diverticula are neither inflamed or infected, the condition is known as diverticulosis. Research reveals that 80 percent of patients with diverticulosis present with no symptoms (Persons, 2019). Thus, since there is no symptom, treatments are unnecessary. However, in worse cases, diverticulosis is known to trigger gastrointestinal symptoms such as abdominal pain and bloating. When this occurs, the condition is termed SUDD (symptomatic uncomplicated diverticular disease). When diverticulosis develops into SUDD, there's a 4% chance that it might further worsen to diverticulitis.

Once diverticula appears, they never really disappear again unless they are removed through surgery. As a result, diverticulosis could last a lifetime if untreated. Albeit, the condition is manageable with some dietary adjustments. With adequate treatment, symptoms of diverticulosis, including bleeding and pain, could abate within a couple of days. But it's worth noting that symptoms could persist or worsen in the event of severe illnesses or complications. People who consume lots of fiber in their day-to-day diets have a lower susceptibility to developing diverticular diseases. The American Dietetic Association posits that the daily recommended intake of fiber borders between 20 to 35 grams. But not all fibers are good for the body. For diverticulosis, you are better off getting your fiber from grains, fruits, and veggies. Your physician or dietician could also place you on a diet with unprocessed bran or specific fiber products. To improve your daily intake of fiber, undergo the process gradually. Additionally, you should take lots of water to help bowel movements by improving bulk. Doing this will help to reduce pressure when passing the bowel.

Diverticulitis

Diverticulitis only occurs due to infection and inflammation (swelling) in one or multiple diverticula. Meaning, for diverticulitis to occur, one must already have diverticulosis. Fever, nausea, and pain are some of the common symptoms of diverticulitis, among others. Unlike diverticulosis, diverticulitis is a graver condition with potential to become dangerous over time. This condition, however, is treatable. For mild diverticulitis, antibiotics, changes in diet, and enough rest can help to cure symptoms. But recurring or severe diverticulitis may require surgical procedures. In simpler terms, diverticulitis is a pretty serious condition, which could range from microperforations in the diverticula to more severe occurrences. When microperforations occur, the diverticula develops tiny holes, which can potentially empty the contents of the colon into the abdominal cavity.

These perforations stem from the constant strain and pressure caused by the movement of stool via the colon. Sometimes, the diverticula could be outrightly ruptured in the process, leading to graves entering and contaminating the peritoneum—the membrane encasing the abdominal cavity. Ruptures could also stem from abscesses, which are infected diverticula with pus, which could grow and ruin the tissues of the colon. If the abscesses that appear on the colon are tiny and do not exceed the region, they could be cleared up with some antibiotic treatment. Otherwise, they might have to be drained to prevent further complications. Large abscesses present even bigger problems and could worsen the condition due to the risk of the infection leaking out and contaminating the outer region of the colon.

Another complication of diverticulitis is peritonitis, which demands immediate surgical intervention to clean out the abdominal cavity and remove the damaged areas of the colon. Without the necessary surgery, peritonitis is a fatal condition. Fistula is another such condition, presenting as the abnormal connection of tissues between different organs. When a damaged tissue touches a different organ, it could stick there. And when it heals that way, it results in a fistula. When diverticulitis infections spread outside the colon, the tissue of the organ could stick to another nearby organ (bladder, skin, or small intestine). Fistulas commonly form between the bladder and colon, and is more prevalent in men than women. They can result in chronic infections in the urinary tract, which requires surgery to remove the affected area of the colon and the fistula.

An infected diverticula could also lead to scarring, which may result in total or partial blockage of the large intestine. When such intestinal obstruction occurs, it becomes difficult for the colon to manage bowel movement effectively. Hence, emergency surgical interventions are imperative. Partial blockages aren't as dire and won't be treated as emergencies, so surgical interventions can be planned.

Am I at Risk?

Diverticulosis is a common condition in people above the age of 40. It seldom occurs in people below the 30-year-old bracket. According to experts, diverticula are more likely to present as you age, and men are more susceptible to the condition than women. Studies also reveal that diverticulosis could occur as a result of genetics (Coble, et al. 2017), meaning that you are more likely to develop diverticula if any of your siblings or parents have them.

Some other risk factors include the following:

- Age: As mentioned earlier, your susceptibility to diverticulosis increases as you age.

- Gender: Males are more likely to develop diverticula than females.

- Weight: A severe case of obesity increases your chances of developing diverticula and contracting diverticulitis.

- Diet: If you regularly consume diets that are low on fiber and steer clear of grains, breads, legumes and beans, nuts, vegetables, and fruits, you are more likely to develop diverticula. Additionally, a diet high in red meat and fat can contribute to the formation of diverticula.

- Smoking: Cigarette smokers have a much higher likelihood than nonsmokers of developing both diverticula and diverticulitis.

- Lack of exercise: Indulging in vigorous exercises tends to decrease the risk of diverticulitis.

- Medications: Certain drugs have been shown to improve the likelihood of developing diverticulitis. These drugs usually come in the form of opioids, steroids, and nonsteroidal anti-inflammatories, such as Aleve (naproxen sodium), and ibuprofen like Motrin IB, Advil, among others.

Chapter 2

Causes and Symptoms of Diverticulitis

It is unclear why diverticula forms, and many experts have varying opinions on the subject. For some, strains or muscle spasms, especially during bowel movements, is the key reason for pressure buildup in the colon, which pushes against the inner lining. Formerly, many experts believed that inadequate consumption of fiber, which can be found in vegetables and fruits, legumes, and grains, can result in diverticulosis. However, recent inquiries into the subject are yet to reveal any clear relationship between diverticula and the consumption of fiber-rich foods.

Another potential theory is that, although unsure of the original triggers of diverticulitis, infection tends to begin as a result of the bacteria content in stools that are pushed into the diverticula. A different theory posits that the walls of the diverticula are subject to erosions from constant and increased pressure levels in the walls of the colon.

Symptoms of Diverticulitis

Although diverticulitis isn't known to result in bothersome symptoms, people tend to report any of the following conditions:

- Constipation
- Mild abdominal cramps
- Tenderness over the affected area
- Bloating or swelling

Bear in mind that presenting with one or more of the symptoms mentioned above isn't necessarily an indication that you suffer from diverticulosis. These symptoms are quite common and present in several gastrointestinal disorders ranging from stomach ulcers to inflammatory bowel diseases to irritable bowel syndrome to gallstones to celiac disease to appendicitis.

How Diverticulitis Is Diagnosed

Since symptoms of diverticulitis do not readily present in many people, the condition is usually discovered when the patient is being screened for polyps or evaluated for other conditions. Gastroenterologists can easily locate and reveal diverticula in the colon using a procedure that requires a tiny camera attached to the end of a lighted, flexible tube that is inserted into the rectum. Another procedure that can be used is sigmoidoscopy in which a short tube is used to probe the lower areas of the colon and the rectum alone. For colonoscopy procedures, a longer tube is used and the whole colon is examined. However, the discovery of diverticulosis isn't limited to gastrointestinal procedures alone, and can also be discovered via imaging tests such as barium x-rays and computer tomography (CT) scan.

How Is Diverticulitis Treated?

When diverticula develops on the colon, they don't tend to occur on their own. For most patients, the symptoms never present and no treatments are necessary. However, when the condition is accompanied by symptoms, such as constipation, bloating, bleeding, and abdominal pain, your doctor could place you on a diet with high fiber content. The choice of diet is meant to soften stools and make them easier to pass. According to daily requirements, it's advised that we consume about 20 to 35 grams of fibre, even though many people only ever consume about half of the said amount daily.

The easiest method of improving fiber intake is to consume more grains, vegetables, and fruits. Some examples of foods with high, healthy fiber content include lima beans, broccoli, apples, squash, kidney beans, pears, and baked beans. Alternatively, your doctor could recommend fiber supplements such as polycarbophil, methylcellulose, or psyllium. These products tend to come in different forms like wafers, powders, or pills. Supplemental fiber products work like high-fiber foods, helping to soften and bulk up stool, making bowel movements easier and less strenuous. Your doctor could also prescribe some medication to reduce the level of colon spasms, which can result in discomfort and abdominal cramping.

Chapter 3

What Is the Role of Food in the Development of Diverticulitis?

The formation of diverticula in the body may be linked to the kind of food we eat. Diverticulosis is a more prominent condition in areas of the industrialized western world than in non-industrialized western areas. This difference is largely tied to the diet and levels of physical activities of both sides. As a region climbs the ladder of industrialization, the susceptibility of its inhabitants to diverticulitis increases. Bear in mind that as much as 15 percent of people suffering from diverticulosis will contract diverticulitis. The main lifestyle risk factors that contribute to the development of diverticulitis are a diet with low fiber content, high fat content, and rich in red meat. Problematic habits, like smoking and the relative lack of exercise, also factor in.

Can Nutrition be Used to Manage Diverticulitis?

As at the time of this writing, the diet of patients suffering from acute episodes of mild uncomplicated diverticulitis tends to have little to no modifications or restrictions. However, some physicians are likely to place patients on clear liquid diets for a couple of days. After the period of examination, if the patients experience relief, they are returned to their regular diets. On the other hand, patients that are hospitalized due to diverticulitis will likely be placed on bowel rest with IV hydration and/or nutrition, or on a clear liquid diet depending on the duration and severity of their symptoms.

When it comes to managing patients with diverticulitis for the long-term, studies posit that a switch to vegetarian diets or an increase in the intake of fiber-rich diets could help to decrease the risk of diverticulitis in the long run. A common erroneous belief pertaining to diverticulitis is that patients with the condition are better off avoiding corn, nuts, seeds, and popcorn. Albeit, a study of 47,000 men showed that the development of diverticulitis in no way ties in with the consumption of those foods. In addition, consuming caffeine and alcohol could not be connected to the development of any diverticular condition.

Stages of Diverticulitis

According to the Hinchey classification, diverticulitis can be classified into four different stages, namely:

- First stage: The initial stage is characterized by diverticulitis with mesenteric abscess, localized pericolic, or phlegmon. At this stage, there are abscesses or inflammatory masses in the folds of the small intestine or the fat that surrounds the colon.

- Second stage: The second stage involves diverticulitis with retroperitoneal abscess, intra-abdominal, or walled-off pelvic. At this stage, the abscesses of infected fluid or pus are walled off in the region in the intra-abdominal space or just outside of the peritoneum.

- Third stage: This stage is characterized by perforated diverticulitis that result in generalized purulent peritonitis. At this stage, the inflammation has released pus into the abdomen and the abscesses have exploded.

- Fourth stage: The fourth stage involves the rupture of the diverticula into the peritoneal cavity alongside fecal contamination that results in generalized fecal peritonitis. At this stage, the abscess has ruptured into the peritoneal cavity. This rupture has resulted in an infection caused by the introduction of feces into the peritoneal cavity.

Chapter 4

Why Should You Implement a FODMAP Diet?

When the term, "low-FODMAP diet" is used, it usually refers to a diet with restrictions on certain sugars, which could trigger distress in the digestive system. The diet was developed for and targeted at people suffering from SIBO (small intestinal bacterial overgrowth) and IBS (irritable bowel syndrome). It helps them to decipher the problematic foods in their regular diets, as well as the foods that help abate their symptoms. Unlike some diets, the low-FODMAP diet is only a temporary fix, which must be discussed with and agreed to by your doctor. Medical consultation is necessary because the diet eliminates many foods and cannot be continued for longer periods as a result. It is more of a brief process of discovery of problematic foods.

FODMAP is an acronym for fermentable oligosaccharides, disaccharides, monosaccharides and polyols. The term refers to short-chain carbohydrates or sugars with strong digestive resistance. Rather than getting absorbed into the bloodstream, FODMAPs get to the far end of the intestines where the majority of gut bacteria can be found. Conversely, the gut bacteria makes use of these carbohydrates as fuel to produce hydrogen gas, as well as certain digestive symptoms, especially in sensitive people. FODMAPs could also pull liquid into the intestines and thus, can result in a case of diarrhea.

How Low-FODMAP Diets Work

The low-FODMAP diet entails three steps of restrictive dieting:

1. The first step involves eating some foods, especially ones with low FODMAP levels.

2. The second step involves a gradual reintroduction to the restricted foods to decipher the ones that cause the most digestive problems.

3. Lastly, once the problematic foods and their respective symptoms are discovered, you can choose to restrict or avoid them totally, while continuing to enjoy every other food as normal.

It's advisable to follow the first step of the low-FODMAP diet for a period of two to six weeks, maximum. During this period, your symptoms will likely decrease. For people with SIBO, it will help to reduce insanely high amounts of bacteria in the intestinal tract. Then, after a period of three days, you can reintroduce a high FODMAP food into your diet, one after the other, and watch carefully for disturbing symptoms. If any one high FODMAP food triggers some symptoms, it's best you avoided that food in the long-term. So, for the big question, you should implement a low-FODMAP diet because it helps you to understand how your system interacts with the foods you eat, the best food for digestive health, and the foods to avoid that cause digestive distresses.

The 4 FODMAPS Explained

Fermentable

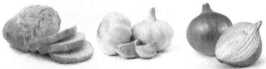

Oligosaccharides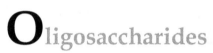

Carbohydrates in the first FODMAP includes **fructans**, which is a combination of oligosaccharides and inulin, and galactooligosaccharides, which can be found in some of the most popular carbohydrates, such as **rye, wheat, fruits, legumes, and vegetables**. Just because FODMAPs should be consumed in a low quantity does not mean that they are necessarily unhealthy types of food; it's just food your body may not accommodate too well.

Disaccharides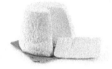

Dairy, or lactose-ingredient products, are considered the main disaccharide that forms a part of FODMAP. It includes foods such as **yogurt, milk, and certain types of cheeses, particularly soft cheese.** You may have heard about people being diagnosed with lactose intolerance, which is the body's direct response to sensitivity to the FODMAP disaccharide.

Monosaccharides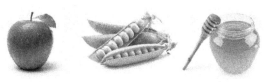

Even though natural sugar is recommended above processed sugar and always will be, some people can be extremely sensitive to fructose, which can be found in different types of **fruit, agave nectar, and the most healing ingredient of all, honey.**

And...

Polyols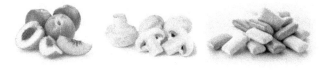

The final FODMAP includes carbohydrates, such as **sorbitol, xylitol, and mannitol,** all of which can be found in sugar-free gum and sweeteners. It can also be found in some fruits and vegetables in small quantities

What Foods Can I Eat on a Low-FODMAP Diet?

Foods that cause distressing symptoms vary across people. However, the key to reducing SIBO and IBS symptoms is avoiding high FODMAP foods that tend to aggravate your gut. These include the following:

- Certain vegetables like **garlic, asparagus, artichokes, and onions.**
- Wheat-based products like **bread, crackers, and cereals.**
- Several fruits, including: **peaches, pears, cherries, and apples.**
- Dairy-based products like **ice cream, yogurt, and milk.**
- Legumes like **lentils and beans.**

Instead, you can include the following low-FODMAP foods into your diet:

- Some cheeses like **cheddar, feta, Camembert, and brie.**
- Fruits like **pineapple, strawberries, grapes, blueberries, and oranges.**
- **Almond milk**
- Vegetables such as **zucchinis, eggplants, cucumbers, potatoes, and tomatoes.**
- Grains such as **oats, quinoa, and rice.**

Who Should Use a Low-FODMAP Diet?

A low-FODMAP diet is intended to be a source of therapy for people with SIBO and IBS. According to studies, this dieting type can reduce up to 86 percent of symptoms in people. Also, since the diet can prove challenging during the first and most restrictive of its three phases, it's imperative that you work under the guidance of a dietician, nutritionist, or doctor. These medical personnel will ensure that you maintain adequate nutrition at all times, and follow the plan correctly, which is necessary for success.

If you are underweight or struggle with weight maintenance, you shouldn't embark on a low-FODMAP diet alone and without medical advice. The low-FODMAP diet cannot be used to achieve weight loss, although the program can alter your weight and cause you to shed some pounds due to its restrictive nature. So, if your weight is already low, losing more would be dangerous.

Benefits of a Low-FODMAP Diet

Patients with IBS (irritable bowel syndrome) are often the case study for low-FODMAP diets. The condition is a widespread digestive problem that presents with symptoms such as constipation, diarrhea, bloating, fast, and stomach cramps. Around 14 percent of the United States population suffer from IBS, and most go undiagnosed. So far, the cause of IBS isn't well-defined, but there are strong connections suggesting that diets play a significant role. Stress is also known to be a key component. According to some studies, up to 75% of people suffering from IBS can gain from a low-FODMAP diet. In several cases, these people went on to experience major reductions in symptoms, as well as major improvements in their overall quality of life.

An emerging area of study in nutrition and diets revolves around the use of a low-FODMAP diet for treating diverticula pain or diverticulitis. Although the said diet was targeted at alleviating symptoms associated with irritable bowel syndrome (IBS), there are several different research studies that suggest that a low-FODMAP diet could help people with diverticula as well (Coppola, 2020). This is because an increase in the internal pressure of the colon can spark irritation and pain in the diverticula. The presence of lots of gases and pressure in the bowel have a higher likelihood of pushing against the mucosa of the colon, thereby creating pockets or further enlarging the pockets that already exist.

As a result, a diet with lower fermentable carbs, like the low-FODMAP diet, could prove to be useful in lowering the outcome of symptoms in patients with diverticula or diverticulitis. Albeit, the area of research suggesting the use of this diet type is relatively new. Hence, the adoption of a low-FODMAP diet for the treatment of diverticulosis or diverticulitis must be permitted by a registered dietician or physician.

A low-FODMAP diet could also prove beneficial for dealing with other FGIDs (functional gastrointestinal disorders), which is a term encompassing many different digestive issues. Additionally, there is evidence that suggests that low-FODMAP diets can be used to treat people suffering from IBDs (inflammatory bowel diseases), such as ulcerative colitis and Crohn's disease. Below are some other benefits the you stand to gain by adopting a low-FODMAP diet:

- Improvement in quality of life: People with irritable bowel syndromes tend to experience a reduction in the quality of life, as well as severe digestive symptoms until undergoing a low-FODMAP diet. Fortunately, there are studies that have discovered a link between low-FODMAP diets and improvements in general quality of life. Also, there is some evidence revealing a connection between increment in energy levels and a low-FODMAP diet in people suffering from IBS. However, this finding needs to be supported by placebo-controlled research.

- Reduction in digestive symptoms: The digestive symptoms of IBS patients can vary across patients, ranging from bowel urgency to flatulence to reflux to stomach pain to bloating to bowel urgency. Stomach pain is usually the hallmark of irritable bowel syndrome, and bloating has been discovered to impact over 80 percent of patients with IBS. It goes without saying that the symptoms of IBS can be quite debilitating. A study reported that patients with IBS reportedly appeared to be willing to give up, on average, up to 25 percent of the remainder of their years to enjoy symptom-free lives (Drossman, et al. 2010).

Luckily, a low-FODMAP diet has been shown to be key in tackling symptoms like bloating and stomach pain. The results from four research studies were conclusive in stating that the odds of improving symptoms like bloating and stomach pain by following a low-FODMAP diet are 75% and 81% greater, respectively (Gutcare, 2020). Many other similar studies have also posited that the diet could help in dealing with diarrhea, constipation, and flatulence.

For a complete guide to the Low-Fodmap diet *check out my book!*
Included you'll find 101 recipes and a detailed list of foods to avoid and eat + again, a 28-day eating plan

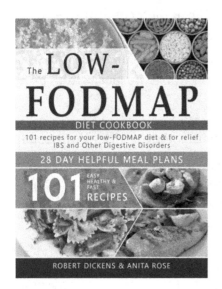

Low FODMAP diet cookbook
101 Easy, healthy & fast recipes for yours low-FODMAP diet + 28 days helpful meal plans

FAQs

What happens in the body when I eat FODMAP foods?

FODMAPs are the chemical construct of foods, which are easily broken down by intestinal bacteria. These foods tend to draw more water into the gut and result in the increased production of gas which, in turn, leads to distension and bloating. Furthermore, they influence the muscle contraction in your gut. As such, people suffering from diverticulosis, diverticulitis, and IBS may experience gastrointestinal discomforts, including diarrhea, abdominal pain, and constipation. People without the aforementioned conditions may consume FODMAPs without concern, but those with any of the above conditions are better off with a low-FODMAP diet.

When cooking, do FODMAPs break down into more digestible forms?

Studies reveal that methods of food preservation, like canning and acidic preservations like pickling tend to heighten the FODMAP content of foods. When legumes are canned, such as chickpeas and lentils, water-soluble FODMAPs are drained from the legumes into the brine they are preserved in. As such, those on a low-FODMAP diet must discard the brine mixture and wash canned legumes before consuming them. When artichokes are pickled, the gradual drain of FODMAPs, as well as the combination of acid can greatly impact the fructans content of the artichokes. Fructans are a form of carbohydrates with poor absorption, which classify as a FODMAP.

Although it's quite possible that immensely high temperatures could affect, and perhaps, break down FODMAPs in foods, it's worth noting that the extent of such a reaction tends to differ greatly across the type of food being cooked. Also, the temperature of cooking as well as several other cooking conditions could play roles in the decomposition of FODMAPs. Put simply, it is quite difficult to accurately predict the effectiveness of cooking in lowering the value of FODMAPs in any given food. Hence, it isn't recommended to use cooking to lower the FODMAP content of foods until more research is carried out to certify otherwise. As at the time of this writing, the best and more reliable course of approach is to stick to low-FODMAP foods and ingredients when cooking.

How can I flavor my food without using garlic, onions, of both?

Onions and garlic classify as high-FODMAP herbs because of their fructan component. Hence, they are unsuitable for use in a low-FODMAP diet. Albeit, since these herbs are widely used in flavoring and cooking in general, it can be quite challenging for most people to cook without them. But there is a way around this hurdle. You can use both herbs to flavor your foods without increasing the FODMAP content of your dish. Bear in mind that FODMAPs are insoluble in oil, hence, ingredients like garlic-infused oils can be used to add flavor to your meals. To make the infused oil, all you have to do is sauté a couple of whole garlic pieces. Neither smash nor finely chop the garlic. Just sauté them whole in oil for a minute or two, until the flavor of the herb seeps into the oil. Afterwards, take out and discard the remnants of garlic, because the clove still retains its high FODMAP content.

Why do certain dried fruits have higher FODMAP value than their fresh fruit alternative, which classify as low-FODMAPs?

To prepare dried fruits, fresh fruits are dehydrated to remove their liquid content. During this process, the sugar content in the fruits are concentrated, as well as the FODMAPs that are usually present in the fresh fruit prior. Experts have also revealed the presence of fructans in dried fruits, which aren't present in fresh fruits of the same crop. Also, dried fruits usually undergo substantial shrinkage in comparison to the real sizes of their fresh fruit alternatives. As such, you can easily eat more dried fruits without realizing it. Thus goes to show why it's imperative to have serving sizes. Consult your dietician for the right servings for any type of dried fruits instead of relying on your satisfaction levels.

Some dried fruits, such as cranberries typically have a higher FODMAP value when they are consumed in larger serving sizes. For smaller servings, dried cranberries have relatively low FODMAP levels and can be tolerated by people with irritable bowel syndrome.

What can I do if low-FODMAP foods still present gut symptoms?

Avoid large servings of any food that triggers gut symptoms similar to diverticulosis and diverticulitis. Ensure to limit your intake of dried fruits and fruit juices to safer quantities as well. Foods that classify as low-FODMAPs, especially fruits, can be tolerated by many people with diverticulitis and diverticulosis. Provided they stick to the right serving sizes recommended by their nutritionist or physician, of course. There are several other dietary components capable of inducing different reactions, including gut symptoms, among a limited amount of people. If your symptoms don't abate despite sticking to a particular low-FODMAP diet, consider consulting your nutritionist or physician to discuss possible intolerances.

Do meats have low-FODMAP values?

Difference sources of animal proteins like eggs, fish, chicken, and meat typically present as low-FODMAP foods because they have little to no carbohydrate content. Albeit, it's imperative to steer clear of ingredients with high FODMAP content, which can be added during the preparation of the aforementioned foods. Those ingredients could include gravies, bread crumbs, marinades, garlic, sauces, and onions.

Do fats and oils have high FODMAP content? What's the difference between using oils like coconut oil and olive oil?

Usually, fats and oils classify as low-FODMAP foods because they have little to no carb values. Although, it's imperative to understand that fats and oils can influence gut motility and, in the event of high consumption, can result in several gut symptoms in some individuals. You also have to be wary of oil-based condiments and sauces, such as aioli and salad dressings, as they may contain ingredients with high FODMAP values, such as onions and garlic. To be on the safe side, always peruse the ingredients lists of such products before consuming them.

To lower the risk of chronic diseases as well as improve overall well-being, experts recommend decreasing the intake of fats and oils with high saturated fats content, such as coconut oil, palm oil, and butter.

Can I go on a low-FODMAP diet for life?

Absolutely not! The purpose of low-FODMAP diets is to improve gut health and help reintroduce some foods into your regular diet over a certain timeframe. The advisable period for practicing low-FODMAP diets ranges from two to six weeks. By the end of the given period, your progress will be reviewed by your physician or dietician. Afterwards, s/he will advise you on the foods to take, as well as how much of them to take, and how to gradually introduce them into your day-to-day diet. Keep in mind that low-FODMAP diets are typically tailored to your needs, so there's no fixed template.

Following the early diet restrictions, many people tend to return to their regular eating habits, with only a couple of foods with high-FODMAP values needing to be consumed in controlled amounts. Studies in recent times show that sticking to a restrictive low-FODMAP diet in the long run can lead to the depletion of a certain amount of beneficial gut bacteria. As a result, it's recommended to not continue with an unnecessarily restrictive low-FODMAP diet. Instead, you should consider seeking specialist advice from a dietician to appropriately reintroduce foods with FODMAP into your day-to-day diet.

Chapter 5

Diverticula Meal Planning

The Clear Liquid Phase

Mild cases of diverticulitis are treated using nutrition therapy. Usually, the most common approach is to start with a clear liquid diet. This type of diet is a medically indicated protocol aimed at alleviating severe GI conditions. The clear liquid diet is but a temporary fix and is useful for helping the digestive system rest up and heal. The aim of the program is to keep the body as hydrated as possible, while still consuming all the adequate nutrients required by the body.

The clear liquid diet is only helpful for a couple of days at a time. Your dietician or doctor should help you to make plans to transition your system back to your normal diet plans as soon as your symptoms start to dissipate. For people with diabetes, it's best to work with a nutritionist when battling diverticulitis. Doing this will ensure that you get the adequate amount of carbs when the doctor monitors your blood sugar levels.

Components of a Clear Liquid Diet

- Sports drinks
- Gelatin
- Broth
- Jell-O
- Honey
- Water
- Ice chips
- Fruit juices without pulp
- Coffee or tea without cream
- Ice pops without bits of pulp or fruit

Clear Liquid Diet Food Plan

When undergoing the clear liquid diet, follow a plan like the one below:

This is only an example, check the components list or follow meal plan at page 36

	Breakfast	Snack (1)	Lunch	Snack (2)	Dinner
Sweeteners	Honey / sugar Or others			Honey / sugar Or others	
Main course	One bowl of gelatin	One bowl of gelatin	One bowl of gelatin, and one cup of broth.		One bowl of gelatin, and one cup of broth.
Food & Beverages	A glass of fruit juice (pulp-free variety), and one cup of tea.	One glass of fruit juice (pulp-free variety)	One glass of fruit juice (pulp-free variety), and one glass of water	One cup of tea without dairy One popsicle (pulp-free variety)	One cup of tea without dairy, water, or one glass of fruit juice (pulp-free variety)

The Advantages and Disadvantages of a Clear Liquid Diet

Advantages

A clear liquid diet is relatively easier to follow, because the recipes are simple to make. The program is also cheap so the fear of breaking the bank is eliminated. Clear liquid diets are the usual prescription after medical tests and surgery, so they ensure speedy recovery.

Disadvantages

The fun of undertaking a clear liquid diet can quickly wear off, especially when trying it for the first time. So, there's the risk of getting bored over time (although this varies across patients). Since clear liquid diets are restrictive, you will easily feel hungry, as the diet lacks certain calories and nutrients you get from your regular diets.

Guidelines for Undergoing a Clear Liquid Diet

Before starting a clear liquid diet, here are a list of things you should know and be prepared for:

- If your physician or dietician places you on a clear liquid diet before a colonoscopy, endeavor to steer clear of red or purple-colored liquids, as they can interfere with imaging tests. If this detail doesn't influence anything, your physician will alert you.

- As mentioned earlier, clear liquid diets don't contain many calories and nutrients. As such, it should not be used for long (**max 3 days**). Stick to the instructions of your physician or dietician when using the clear liquid diet plan.

- If you have diabetes, it's best to inform your physician or dietician about it. A clear liquid diet can provide diabetic patients with as much as 200g go carbs spread across one day.

    This should help with effective blood sugar management. Carefully watch and track your blood sugar levels and quickly transition back to solid foods as soon as possible.

The Juicing Diet

Juice fasts or juicing diets have proven to be more than the mere fad they were thought to be back in the day. They have gained traction and become mainstream in recent times. There are many people who swear by the juicing diet for many reasons, including their influence on weight loss. Juicing diets revolve around diets that include juices or other clear liquids, such as tea and water. Juice dieting, otherwise known as juice cleansing or juice fasting, aids the body to recover nutrients. The term "juicing" implies the extraction of the liquid content of whole fruits and vegetables. The only thing missing from the juices of vegetables and fruits is the fiber provided by the pulp. Although fiber is key to any healthy diet, it can result in problems for the digestive system if consumed in bulk.

Moreover, the juice from fruits and vegetables is rich in vitamins, phytonutrients, and minerals. When embarking on a juicing diet, the gastrointestinal tract is given the chance to rest and heal. And since the food absorbed isn't in solid form, it allows for easier absorption of nutrients by the digestive system. For many, juicing helps to boost the immune system, shed or manage weight, and flush toxins out of the body.

How the Juicing Diet Works

Before turning to a juicing diet, consult with your dietician or physician. Next, it's imperative that you pick the right recipes and ingredients. It's advisable to go for organic vegetables and fruits since they are lacking in farmyard chemicals like pesticides and fertilizers. Your doctor or dietician should be aware of how long you intend to carry on the diet. Finally, ensure that your choice of fruits and vegetables classify as low-FODMAPs.

Time	Juice
Waking up	8 oz. of hot water with lemon or ginger
Breakfast	Red or orange juice – 16 oz.
Mid-morning snack	Vegetable broth or coconut water – 16 oz.
Lunch	Green juice – 16 oz.
Afternoon snack	Red or yellow juice – 16 oz.
Dinner	Green juice – 16 oz.
Dessert	Orange or purple juice – 16 oz.
Bedtime	Herbal tea

The color of the juices extracted from vegetables and fruits implies that the ingredients in the juices are of a similar color. Meaning, if you consume different colors of juices, you will be getting a broad range of ingredients. For example:

- Yellow juice is rich in pineapple, yellow bell pepper, among other fruits.
- Purple juices contain purple grapes or blueberries.
- Red juices could contain beets or hibiscus.
- Orange juices could contain bits of sweet potatoes.
- Green juices, in several cases, combine vegetables like celery, kale, and cucumber.

Cons of Juicing

As much as juicing seems like the way to go, what with the elimination of problematic fiber, and, hence, a reduction in high-FODMAP, it isn't altogether safe. It could result in side effects, such as constipation, dizziness, diarrhea, and fatigue. These side effects would typically be resolved by the body as it gets used to the new diet. However, if symptoms such as diarrhea (persistent), fainting, low blood pressure, vomiting, and extreme dizziness set in, it's imperative you consult your doctor immediately.

The Low-Residue Diet

A low-residue diet, otherwise known as a low-fiber diet, is typically recommended when one experiences diverticulitis flare-ups. The aim of this diet type is to decrease the volume of the bowels to foster the healing of the infection. Any intake of less than 10 grams of fiber daily can be considered as a low-residue diet when dealing with diverticulitis. For people who have been on this diet plan for an extensive period, your physician or dietician could recommend a multivitamin supplement to be taken daily.

Hopefully, before this phase, your digestive system has been calmed by the clear liquid diet. Once you start to feel normal again, it's best that you transition to a low-residue diet to continue the healing process. The reason for this follow-up dieting technique is to ensure that the fiber consumed daily can be easily digested. Think of the term "low-residue" as the process of going easy on your digestive system. The Recommended Dietary Allowances can be achieved from both low-fiber and low-residue diets if the correct foods are consumed. However, it's worth noting that continuing with a low-fiber diet for a long time can lead to vitamin C or folic acid deficiency.

Below are some low-residue foods to take into cognizance:

- **Fruits**

Cooked or canned foods without seeds or skin

- **Vegetables**

Cooked or canned vegetables without skin

- **Animal-based protein:**

Poultry, fish, and eggs.

- **Beverage**

Vegetable and fruit juices without pulp.

- **Snacks**

Low-fiber cereals, and refined white bread.

- **Dairy**

Yogurt

- **Grains**

Noodles, pasta, and white rice.

Meal Plan for Your Low-Fiber Diet

Below is a sample meal plan for a low-fiber diet:

DAY	Breakfast	Lunch	Dinner
1	Apple juice – ½ cup	Chicken rice soup – one cup	Grape juice – ½ cup
2	Corn flakes – ¾ cup	Lean hamburger – 3 oz.	Chicken breast – 3 oz.
3	White bread – one slice	One White hamburger buns without seeds	One white roll
4	Margarine – one teaspoon	Iceberg lettuce	Margarine – one teaspoon
5	Jelly – 2 tsp.	One cup 2% milk	Mashed potato – ½ cup
6	One cup 2% milk	Fruit cocktail – ½ cup	Cooked green beans – ½ cup
7	Tea/coffee	Fasting	Honeydew melon – ½ cup; tea/coffee

PS: The milk used in any of the meal plans mentioned in this section is the dairy-free variety. Also, a low-fiber diet should only be followed for about two days, after which it should be discontinued. Meaning, the table above is not a weekly template of a low-fiber diet plan, but several alternatives to pick from. Finally, if you must continue the diet for longer than necessary, consult with your doctor or dietician.

General Guidelines for Following a Low-Residue Diet

- Go for canned or cooked fruits and vegetables other than their fresh or raw alternatives. Remember that some fruits and vegetables could lead to gastrointestinal discomforts. Endeavor to steer clear of these foods.
- Stick to the low-fiber guidelines when picking meals. Avoid taking more than two cups of milk or dairy products in one day.
- Add foods like rice products, white bread, and refined cereals to your diet. Steer clear of food products made with whole grain flour, bran, nuts, and seeds.
- Avoid introducing prune juice into your diet.
- When taking meats, ensure they are properly cooked, tender, and ground. Steer clear of dried beans and peas.

Transitional Phase

The transitional phase involves the gradual reintroduction of high-fiber foods into your diet. It is usually the final stage after a clear liquid diet and low-fiber diet. The aim of this phase is to help the body rediscover its rhythm with your regular diet until you can return back with little to no risks gastrointestinal discomforts.

Below are some foods you can incorporate into your diet at this phase:

- **Fruits**

Pear, kale, quinoa, pomegranate, etc.

- **Vegetables**

Cauliflower, chickpeas, sweet potatoes, brussels sprouts, swiss chard, etc.

- **Animal-based protein:**

Poultry (chicken), fish (salmon), and eggs.

- **Other foods include**

Oatmeal, brown rice, granola, steak, tacos, pork loins, pancakes, smoothies, etc.

Below is a meal plan template for all three phases: liquid diet, low-fiber diet, and the transitional phase.

28-Day Meal Plan

Below you will find an eating plan that will guide you through your treatment for 28 days.

This food plan is divided into 4 phases:

For the first 2 days you must only consume liquid foods, without the pulp or lumps, so if you make yourself some juice make sure you filter it well! As mentioned above in this phase we want the whole digestive system to relax and not dispose of solid parts of the food.

In the second phase, we will begin to introduce low fiber foods. The only purpose of this phase is to ensure proper digestion without risking inflammation of the diverticula. This phase will end after eight days.

In the third phase, however, we will reintroduce fiber, so you can go back to eating as before. Remember, however, not to overwork your digestion by eating too much, and every now and then drink a herbal tea to relax and cleanse the intestines.

In the last phase, we are going to introduce the Low-FODMAP diet. As already explained in the previous chapter eating foods low in FODMAP helps to eliminate abdominal bloating, in doing so we would reduce the risk of inflammation of diverticula and we can feel safe eating these recipes.

I remind you that this food plan is an indication, you are not required to eat any recipe that you do not like. The important thing is to eat foods compatible with the 4 phases, so take a good look at the recipes and choose the ones you like best!

NB: In these 28 days remember to cut down, it is better to avoid milk and milk derivatives

Scan QR code
To Download **Printable** meal plan

Day 1:
- **Breakfast** - Apple Juice — Pag. 56
- **Lunch** - Vegetable Clear Soup — Pag. 62
- **Dinner** - Vegan Jello — Pag. 68
- **Snack** - Coffee or tea — -

Day 2:
- **Breakfast** - Carrot and Apple Juice — Pag. 55
- **Lunch** - Japanese Clear Soup — Pag. 66
- **Dinner** - Green Smoothie Popsicles — Pag. 71
- **Snack** - Coffee or tea — -

Day 3:
- **Breakfast** - Greek Yogurt Oatmeal Pancake — Pag. 78
- **Lunch** - Chicken Sour Cream Enchiladas — Pag. 82
- **Dinner** - Cauliflower Rice — Pag. 90
- **Snack** - Banana Bread + tea or coffee — Pag. 99

Day 4:
- **Breakfast** - Greek Yogurt Oatmeal Pancake — Pag. 78
- **Lunch** - Spaghetti Sauce With Ground Turkey — Pag. 93
- **Dinner** - Gluten-free Crustless Pizza — Pag. 83
- **Snack** - Banana Bread + tea, coffee or smoothie — Pag. 99

Day 5:
- **Breakfast** - Almond Meal Blueberry Muffins + beverage of your choice — Pag. 77
- **Lunch** - Sweet Potato Gnocchi — Pag. 94
- **Dinner** - BBQ Beef Stir-Fry — Pag. 89
- **Snack** – banana or fruit juice — -

Day 6:
- **Breakfast** - Almond Meal Blueberry Muffins + beverage of your choice — Pag. 77
- **Lunch** - Chicken Fingers — Pag. 81
- **Dinner** - Tomato Pasta — Pag. 86
- **Snack** - banana + tea, coffee or smoothie — -

Day 7:
- **Breakfast** - Easy Peanut Butter Cookies with tea or coffee — Pag. 101
- **Lunch** - Tomato Pasta — Pag. 86
- **Dinner** - Sweet Potato Gnocchi — Pag. 94
- **Snack** - Oatmeal Peanut Butter Balls with tea or coffee — Pag. 104

Day 8:
- **Breakfast** - Banana Bread with beverage of your choice — Pag. 99
- **Lunch** - Green Curry Tofu Rice — Pag. 121
- **Dinner** - Marinated Pear and Fennel With Chickpeas — Pag. 124
- **Snack** - Oatmeal Peanut Butter Balls with tea or coffe — Pag. 104

Day 9:
- **Breakfast** - Apple Pie Oatmeal — Pag. 109
- **Lunch** - Chicken Breast With Kabocha and Kale — Pag. 117
- **Dinner** - Brussels Sprouts and Sweet Potato Hash — Pag. 133
- **Snack** – yogurt — -

Day 10:
- **Breakfast** - Banana Buckwheat Pancakes and Compote — Pag. 110
- **Lunch** - Green Curry Tofu Rice — Pag. 121
- **Dinner** - Parmesan Cauliflower With Chickpeas — Pag. 137
- **Snack** - choose the snak you prefer — -

Day 11:
- **Breakfast** - Black Bean Spinach Quesadilla — Pag. 111
- **Lunch** - Flat-Belly Salad — Pag. 120
- **Dinner** - Rainbow Veggie Chili — Pag. 138
- **Snack** – tea, coffe or smoothie with some cookies — -

Day 12:
- **Breakfast** - Savory Cheese Oatmeal — Pag. 115
- **Lunch** - Lentil Soup — Pag. 123
- **Dinner** - Greek Chicken Pasta — Pag. 135
- **Snack** - choose the snak you prefer — -

Day 13:
- **Breakfast** - Apple Pie Oatmeal — Pag. 109
- **Lunch** - Hearty Vegetable Curry — Pag. 122
- **Dinner** - Salmon Quinoa and Roasted Brussel Sprouts — Pag. 141
- **Snack** - choose the snak you prefer — -

Day 14:
- **Breakfast** - Greek Yogurt Oatmeal Pancake + coffe or tea — Pag. 78
- **Lunch** - Cauliflower Rice — Pag. 90
- **Dinner** - Sweet Potato With White Bean Bake — Pag. 145
- **Snack** - tea, coffe or smoothie with some cookies — -

Day 15:
- **Breakfast** - Banana Buckwheat Pancakes and Compote — Pag. 110
- **Lunch** - Spicy Red Lentil Soup — Pag. 125
- **Dinner** - Grilled Zucchini Hummus — Pag. 136
- **Snack** - Energy Bars — Pag. 184

Day 16:
- **Breakfast** - tea, coffe or smoothie with some cookies — -
- **Lunch** - Sweet Potato Chili — Pag. 127
- **Dinner** - Roasted Pork Loin With Apple Jus — Pag. 139
- **Snack** - Yogurt With Pumpkin Granola — Pag. 151

Day 17:
- **Breakfast** - Chocolate Cherry Egg White Oatmeal — Pag. 112
- **Lunch** - Flat-Belly Salad — Pag. 120
- **Dinner** - Grilled Zucchini Hummus — Pag. 136
- **Snack** - choose the snak you prefer — -

Day 18:
- **Breakfast** - Savory Cheese Oatmeal — Pag. 115
- **Lunch** - Flat-Belly Salad — Pag. 120
- **Dinner** - Sheet Pan Salmon — Pag. 142
- **Snack** - Yogurt — -

Day 19:
- **Breakfast** - tea, coffe or smoothie with some cookies — -.
- **Lunch** - Spiced Tomato Lentil Soup — Pag. 126
- **Dinner** - Parmesan Cauliflower With Chickpeas — Pag. 137
- **Snack** - Energy Bars — Pag. 184

Day 20:
- **Breakfast** - Cinnamon French Toast — Pag. 113
- **Lunch** - Chicken Breast With Kabocha and Kale — Pag. 117
- **Dinner** - Flank Steak Tacos — Pag. 134
- **Snack** - Banana Nuts Overnight Oats — Pag. 149

Day 21:
- **Breakfast** - Cinnamon French Toast — Pag. 113
- **Lunch** - Spicy Red Lentil Soup — Pag. 125
- **Dinner** - Superfast Asparagus — Pag. 144
- **Snack** - Kale and Pear Smoothie — Pag. 150

Day 22:
- **Breakfast** - Banana Porridge — Pag. 154
- **Lunch** - Corn Salad — Pag. 162
- **Dinner** - Bolognese — Pag. 169
- **Snack** - Summer Popsicle — Pag. 181

Day 23:
- **Breakfast** - Pineapple, Strawberry, Raspberry Smoothie — Pag. 156
- **Lunch** - Chicken Wrap — Pag. 164
- **Dinner** - Vegetable Fried Rice — Pag. 171
- **Snack** - Orange Biscuits with coffe or tea — Pag. 182

Day 24:
- **Breakfast** - Banana Oatcakes — Pag. 155
- **Lunch** - Quiche in Ham Cups — Pag. 165
- **Dinner** - Feta Meatball — Pag. 173
- **Snack** - Quinoa Muffins with coffe or tea — Pag. 179

Day 25:
- **Breakfast** - Crepes and Berries — Pag. 158
- **Lunch** - Rice & Zucchini Slice — Pag. 167
- **Dinner** - Minestrone — Pag. 170
- **Snack** - Chocolate Peanut Butter Energy Bites — Pag. 180

Day 26:
- **Breakfast** - Egg Wraps — Pag. 153
- **Lunch** - Tomato and Green Bean Salad — Pag. 161
- **Dinner** - Vegan Curry — Pag. 176
- **Snack** - Pineapple, Strawberry, Raspberry Smoothie — Pag. 156

Day 27:
- **Breakfast** - Banana Porridge — Pag. 154
- **Lunch** - Feta, Chicken, and Pepper Sandwich — Pag. 166
- **Dinner** - Gnocchi — Pag. 175
- **Snack** - Coconut Bites — Pag. 183

Day 28:
- **Breakfast** - Crepes and Berries — Pag. 158
- **Lunch** - Pesto Noodles — Pag. 163
- **Dinner** - Bolognese — Pag. 169
- **Snack** - Blueberry, Lime, and Coconut Smoothie — Pag. 157

Chapter 6

Creating the Perfect Shopping List

A diet food list for diverticular diseases with several decades of fiber-rich foods, clear liquid foods, and low-fiber foods helps people with diverticulitis know what's safe to eat at any one time. The foods are categorized into three, namely:

Acute Phase Foods

This category comprises of foods for a clear liquid diet:

- Dry toast
- Jell-O without fruit
- Fruit juices without pulp
- Plain saltine crackers
- Chicken or beef broth
- Water, tea, or coffee (without dairy)
- Popsicles or ice chips (pulp-free)

Recovery Phase Foods

This category is for foods for a low-fiber diet:

- Yogurt
- Toast and soft or hard boiled eggs
- Well cooked vegetables (skinned)
- vegetable soup
- Low-fiber cereals
- Canned fruits (pulp-free)
- Juices (pulp-free)
- Peanut butter
- Macaroni, rice, and plain noodles
- Fish, meat, and poultry

Prevention Foods

This category is for reintroducing fiber into your diet:

- Fish, poultry, meat
- Wild rice
- Brown rice
- Vegetables
- Fruits with pulp
- Cereals and bread (whole grain variety)
- Dried beans and lentils
- **All foods with low-FODMAP**

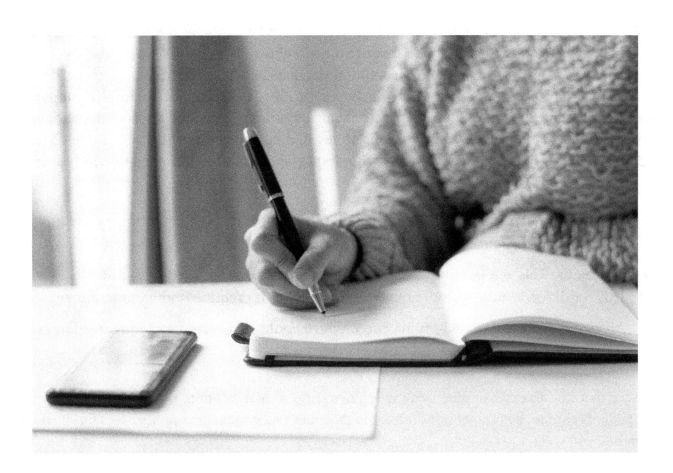

Chapter 6

Myths About Diverticular Diseases

All diverticular diseases require treatment:

Patients tend to confuse diverticulitis with diverticulosis. While both conditions share a common umbrella as diverticular diseases, they are distinct in and of themselves. Hence, while diverticulosis will typically not require treatments, as it presents no symptoms, diverticulitis is quite serious and could require surgical intervention. Diverticulosis is a condition that happens due to the presence of diverticula on the walls of the intestines. They are quite a common condition, with up to 60 percent of the populace having diverticula by the age of 69. At 80, up to 80 percent of people have diverticulosis. What's more, the condition is usually discovered by chance during a colonoscopy exam. In fact, many people live their lives without knowing they have diverticulosis. Alone, by themselves, diverticula pose little to no cause for alarm.

Think of diverticulosis like having freckles. It's fine until it becomes a mole. Only then is it a problem. Experts rarely ever attend to cases of diverticulosis, except cases where the diverticula causes bleeding or won't stop bleeding. On the other hand, diverticulitis develops due to perforations, inflammation, or infections happening in the diverticula. It could also be due to rupturing of diverticula or as a result of bacteria infection. Stool contains bacteria, which could be harmful to the body when it leaves the intestines and spreads to the surrounding abdominal region. When that happens, there are several different complications that could arise, including:

- Pain: You'd typically experience a painful sensation when eating, drinking, or swallowing. The pain could also be followed by a fever.
- Peritonitis: This is a painful infection in the abdominal cavity, which is potentially fatal. This condition is quite uncommon, though, and doesn't require imminent treatment.
- Abscesses: This is a walled-off infection, which could occur from bacteria infection in the abdominal cavity.

Note that not all cases of diverticulitis require surgical intervention. However, it's imperative that patients contact their physicians (either in the emergency room or primary care) for adequate diagnosis.

People with diverticular diseases can't eat seeds, popcorn, or nuts:

This is one of the most widespread myths about the condition. In fact, it contradicts the usual advice doctors offer to patients to help prevent diverticulitis and diverticulosis. A diet rich in healthy fiber is a better alternative for preventing diverticulitis, and foods like nuts and seeds are fiber-rich items. The idea behind avoiding popcorn, seeds, and nuts was the belief that these foods could easily get lodged in the pockets in the colon. When this happens, the diverticula could rupture or become inflamed; thus, resulting in diverticulitis. However, this idea isn't only faulty but disingenuous altogether. In fact, studies don't suggest any reasons to avoid these foods.

If you suffered from diverticulosis in the past, which grew into diverticulitis, other bouts of diverticulitis afterwards are more susceptible to perforations and can result in peritonitis:

This is erroneous thinking. First of all, the chances of diverticulitis developing in 25 percent of patients with diverticulosis is only 10. Also, for the greater majority, or the remaining 75 percent, diverticulitis is less severe and could require as little as antibiotic medications or a simple outpatient treatment. Studies reveal that a subsequent bout of diverticulitis is most likely going to follow the patterns of the prior bout. Typically, if your body could manage diverticulitis during the first bout, chances are that it's going to manage just fine the next time too. Often, when patients aren't satisfied with this explanation, they question how they can prevent themselves from getting a second bout. Unfortunately, no one can predict or accurately describe why it happens. Not even your doctor. But it can be assumed that constipation and strain or high pressure during bowel movement plays a role. It's advisable to eat foods rich in fiber, stick to healthy foods, and steer clear of constipation.

Diverticulitis and diverticulosis are the same:

No, they're not. Diverticulosis is a condition characterized by the presence of diverticula. Diverticulitis happens because diverticula become infected or inflamed. Take note of the difference in their suffixes too. The "-osis" in medical terminologies describes a medical condition, while "-it is" is used for inflammation or infections.

Consuming red meat leads to diverticular disease:

This is just wrong. There are no known foods that contribute to the development of diverticulitis or diverticulosis in the body. This myth gained traction after a study suggested that vegetarians had less susceptibility to diverticular conditions than non-vegetarians. In a general sense, vegetarians are more likely to consume more fiber-rich foods than their non-vegetarian counterparts. Hence, it's a given that the fiber content of their food is the telling factor, not their abstinence from red meat.

Going on a liquid diet can help to avoid diverticulitis:

As a treatment for acute diverticulitis attacks, your physician could temporarily recommend a liquid diet for you. However, it doesn't mean that a liquid diet can prevent you from developing diverticulitis. Sure, it's imperative for anyone with diverticular disease to stay hydrated by taking in lots of water. But consuming liquids alone can be detrimental to your body, and your colon even, because of the many essential dietary fibre and nutrients you'll miss out on. Consult your gastroenterologists about the type of diet to follow that would best prevent diverticulitis attacks in the future

Will I require a surgical procedure to get my colon removed if I develop diverticulitis?

Although there could be cases where surgery is needed to manage diverticulitis, it wouldn't always be necessary. Diverticulitis is a pretty fascinating condition, because many people with the condition may never get to go under the knife throughout their lifetime. If you experience recurring attacks of diverticulitis, it could be beneficial for you to have the diseased area of your colon surgically removed. It's only in such a case that seeing a medical professional to discuss surgery is necessary. Another situation would be if there is a large perforation in your colon as a result of diverticulitis. Not only is surgery necessary in this case, but it's also an emergency. You are likely to be very sick and require immediate care to get your system back on track.

Supplements Can't Help Prevent Diverticulitis Attacks:

Although there isn't enough evidence to support or completely debunk the idea of preventing diverticulitis by taking supplements, a small body of research suggests a potential connection between some supplements and a reduction in the risks of diverticulitis (Stollman, et al. 2015). One study posited a possible affiliation between low vitamin D levels and an increment in the likelihood of developing diverticulitis. According to the study, a supplement may just prevent the development of diverticulitis in people suffering from vitamin D deficiency. A different study suggested that using a lactobacillus casei DG probiotic supplement may help protect against the recurrence of a diverticulitis attack. Before taking any supplements, ensure to consult with your gastroenterologists to ascertain if the supplements could help to lower the risk of a recurring attack.

If I switch up my diet, will my condition go away or get better?

This is a tricky question because the go-to treatment for diverticular diseases tends to include nutritional therapy. Diverticulitis is a condition that typically plagues the more industrialized regions of the world. It is only becoming more widespread as the world grows and develops into a more industrialized place. The condition stems from the decrement or deficiency of fiber and a corresponding spike in carbohydrates in a diet. It gets worse when it comes to people who experience chronic constipation. Naturally, the deducible cue would be to improve the fiber content in your diet, wouldn't it? That'd be thoughtful, indeed. However, it's not as easy to reverse the damages caused by the condition. Your diverticula aren't going to be magically whisked away, even if you don't know they exist. So, sure, you could do with adding more fiber to your diet and keeping simple carbohydrates at a respectable minimum, but the best you can do is to prevent things from growing worse. To avoid further complications posed by constipation, it's best that you stay properly hydrated.

It is impossible to avoid subsequent diverticulitis attacks after the first one:

Make no mistake, diverticulitis can be a painful condition and, in certain instances, it can result in severe infections that might require surgical interventions to take out a diseased part of your bowel. With this in mind, it makes sense for people who have experienced the condition to be prepared to do anything to prevent a recurrence. If you are dealing with recurring bouts of diverticulitis attacks, it's advisable to consult your gastroenterologists. They should be able to talk you through the recent studies on the subject, as well as the medications used to manage IBD (inflammatory bowel disease), which could lower the risk of recurring bouts. A recent study posits that combining several medications, including a lactobacillus supplement could help to ward off recurrent diverticulitis attacks.

Diverticular diseases can be prevented:

The route to knowing the prevention of a condition lies in knowing how the said condition came about. Several studies suggest that more than half of the adult population above the age of 50 have diverticula on the colon. What's more, the risk of having diverticula increases with age. It was this logic that led researchers to believe that diverticulosis could be prevented by avoiding constipation. However, recent inquiries into the subject have revealed that constipation or not, diverticulosis cannot be helped. In summary, while diverticular diseases may be relatively impossible to avoid, you can't go wrong with eating a rich, balanced diet high in fiber. Not only would this improve your overall gut health, but it's good for general well-being as well.

Chapter 7

FAQs About Diverticular Diseases

What can I do to avoid diverticular disease?

Once diverticula forms in the colon, it's permanent. There are no known treatments that prevent the formation of other diverticular diseases or complications. Fiber-rich diets can help to improve stool bulk and avoid constipation, but that's as far as it goes. Theoretically, experts believe fiber-rich foods could prevent the formation of diverticula or the development of worse diverticular conditions. People who have a history of diverticular diseases and experience abdominal pains, chills, and inexplicable fever should consult with their physician. Those symptoms could be a potential hint at diverticular complications.

How does diverticula develop?

As we age, the walls of the colon grow thicken. When this happens, diverticula could form as a result of strain or increasing pressure on the colon to pass feces. For instance, a diet with low fiber content can result in small, hard stools, which can cause difficulty in bowel movement. As such, one would need to increase pressure on the bowels to pass. Small stools and fiber deficiency could also result in certain segments of the colon closing off from the rest of the organ during contraction in the segment of colonic muscle. The pressure exerted in the closed-off segments would usually grow higher because the increased pressure is unable to spread evenly across the colon. As time goes by, high pressure in the colon would lead to the inner lining of the intestines to push outward (herniation) in weaker areas of the muscular walls. The sacs or pockets or pouches that develop as a result are known as diverticula.

Can I live a long life if I have diverticulitis?

If diverticulitis becomes severe, you may have to undergo a surgical procedure to have the affected part of your colon removed. It can't be understated that diverticulitis can be a life-changing condition. However, you can still go on to have a normal life with the right treatment and a few alterations to your diet.

Can I eat bananas if I have diverticulitis?

Foods that are rich in fiber, such as bananas, pears, peaches, prunes, tangerines, apples, etcetera are good for diverticulitis patients. Vegetables that are cooked till tender, such as sweet potatoes, broccoli, beets, carrots, lima beans, turnips, asparagus, squash, and mushrooms are also good.

Is diverticular disease a serious condition?

Diverticulitis is the most severe form of diverticular disease. Not only can it lead to severe complications, but it also causes gastrointestinal discomforts. If diverticulitis is left untreated, the condition can grow in the long-term into more complex health issues.

What is diverticular pain like?

Diverticulitis is usually characterized by a sharp pain, sort of like a cramp. The sensation can be felt on the left area of the lower abdomen. Other symptoms to watch out for include diarrhea, constipation, vomiting, nausea, chills, and fever.

Is it bad to take coffee when I have diverticulosis?

When experiencing acute diverticulitis attacks, it's best to go on a low-fiber diet. Steer clear of foods that may result in pain or nausea, such as dairy products, chocolate, spicy foods, and caffeine. When you stop experiencing the symptoms of diverticulitis, you can begin a gradual transition to high-fiber foods.

What is the life expectancy rate for people with diverticulitis?

The mean age of people who have experienced their first attack of diverticulitis is, on estimate, 65 years. As such, patients tend to have an average life expectancy rate of about 14 years.

Does walking help with my diverticulitis?

Studies show that cumulative physical activities may have a decreasing effect on diverticular bleeding and diverticulitis.

What are stools like when one has diverticulitis?

Usually, there are no signs in your stools when you have diverticulitis. However, when the condition worsens, there is likely to be fixation, distortion, or even narrowing around the region of the lower colon. When this happens, stools mat appear to have a pellet or thin-shaped appearance. There could also be an occasional rush of diarrhea and spells of constipation.

Does bed rest improve symptoms of diverticulitis?

People suffering from diverticulitis tend to experience improvement in their symptoms between two to four days after the start of treatment. More than 85 percent of patients tend to recover from symptoms of diverticulitis with some antibiotics, liquid diet, and bed rest. Most of these people never experience a recurrent diverticulitis attack.

Are there foods that cause diverticulitis?

There aren't any specific foods that could trigger diverticulitis attacks or cause diverticulosis. There are also no special diets that prevent diverticular diseases.

MEASUREMENT CONVERSIONS

Volume equivalents (Liquid)

US standard	US Ounces	Metric (approximate)
2 tablespoons	1 fl. Oz.	30 mL
¼ cup	2 fl. Oz.	60 mL
½ cup	4 fl. Oz.	120 mL
1 cup	8 fl. Oz.	240 mL
1½ cup	12 fl. Oz.	355 mL
2 cups or 1 pint	16 fl. Oz.	475 mL
4 cups or 1 quart	32 fl. Oz.	1 L
1 gallon	128 fl. Oz.	4 L

Volume equivalents (Dry)

US standard	Metric (approximate)
⅛ teaspoon	0.5 mL
¼ teaspoon	1 mL
½ teaspoon	2 mL
¾ teaspoon	4 mL
1 teaspoon	5 mL
1 tablespoon	15 mL
¼ cup	59 mL
⅓ cup	79 mL
½ cup	118 mL
⅔ cup	156 mL
¾ cup	177 mL
1 cup	235 mL
2 cups or 1 pint	475 mL
3 cups	700 mL
4 cups or 1 quart	1 L

Oven Temperatures	
Fahrenheit	Celsius (approximate)
250° F	120° C
300° F	150° C
325° F	165° C
350° F	180° C
375° F	190° C
400° F	200° C
425° F	220° C
450° F	230° C

Weight Equivalents	
US Standard	Metric (approximate)
½ ounce	15 g
1 ounce	30 g
2 ounces	60 g
4 ounces	115 g
8 ounces	225 g
12 ounces	340 g
16 ounces or 1 pound	455 g

Chapter 8

Recipes

This section is filled with delicious recipes that you can make at home. There is a wide variety of meals and types of foods. You will not run out of things to cook if you try out these recipes. There is something for everyone.

The best part is that they are all diverticulitis friendly. There are no specific triggers in these recipes, and they are all delicious. They have been divided into categories, so it will be easy to find what you are looking for. It is also easy to find out whether the recipes are vegan or gluten-free. All you have to do is look at the tags. These specific diets have been taken into account, so there is no need to worry if you follow a stricter diet.

Eating for diverticular diseases does not have to be limiting and boring. There are plenty of different meals you can make. It also does not have to be hard to change your diet. Many people quit when they have to change their eating habits because it seems too hard to switch over. Most of these recipes are super easy and quick. There are a few that take a bit longer and are more technical, but you can save those for days when you want to be a little fancy or have more time.

The best strategy is to try a few new recipes each week until you find the ones you really like. It is not expected for you to be making new meals every day. But in the beginning, you will need to experiment, especially if your current diet is filled with diverticulitis triggers. So jump in and find your new favorite, go-to meals.

> The cookbook is divided into 4 parts: the first 3 recipes are aimed at the phases of treatment (clear fluids, low and high fiber). The last part is dedicated to the low-fodmap. I would like to remind you that if you want to delve deeper into the FODMAP diet I have written 2 books about it, and you can find them on **page 187**

Clear Fluids

Breakfast

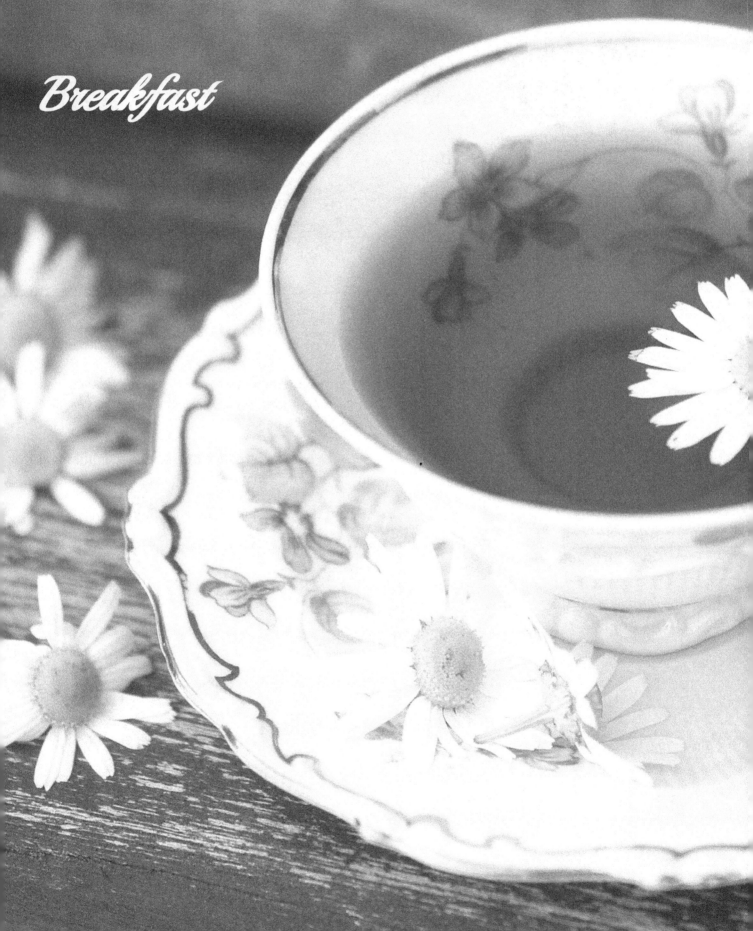

Apple Juice

Cal 82 VEGAN	**Difficulty:** Easy **Preparation time:** 10 minutes **Cook time:** 60 minutes **Servings:** 5

Nutrition per serving (g)

Fat	Saturates	Carbs	Sugars	Protein
0.1	0	21	18.6	0.2

Ingredients

- 3 seeded red apples, keep the peel and core
- ¼ cup white sugar
- 5 cups water

Method

1. Set stove to medium heat and place a saucepan containing water on it. Add the apple cores and peels into the pan.

2. Allow to boil, then reduce the heat to a simmer and stir for about 30 minutes.

3. Discard the peels and cores, and stir in sugar.

4. Set aside to cool for about 30 minutes before serving.

Carrot and Apple Juice

Cal 277 — VEGAN

Difficulty: Easy
Preparation time: 10 minutes
Cook time: -
Servings: 1

Nutrition per serving (g)

Fat	Saturates	Carbs	Sugars	Protein
1.3	0.2	68.6	43.6	4

Ingredients

- 4 carrots, sliced
- ½ inch fresh ginger
- 2 apples, quartered
- 2 stalks celery

Method

1. Using a juicer, process the carrots, apples, and celery in this order. Finally, place ginger in the juicer.

Green Juice

Cal 83 VEGAN	Difficulty: Easy Preparation time: 15 minutes Cook time: - Servings: 4

Nutrition per serving (g)

Fat	Saturates	Carbs	Sugars	Protein
0	0	20	12	2

Ingredients

- 1 bunch curly kale, diced
- 4 celery stalks
- 1 large lemon, quartered
- 2 large apples, cored and chopped
- 1 inch ginger
- 1 large cucumber, sliced into thin vertical strips

Method

1. Clean and prepare the veggies.
2. With a juicer, process the kale, lemon, ginger, cucumbers, apples, and celery in this order.
3. Remove and discard the pulp with a sieve.
4. Serve.

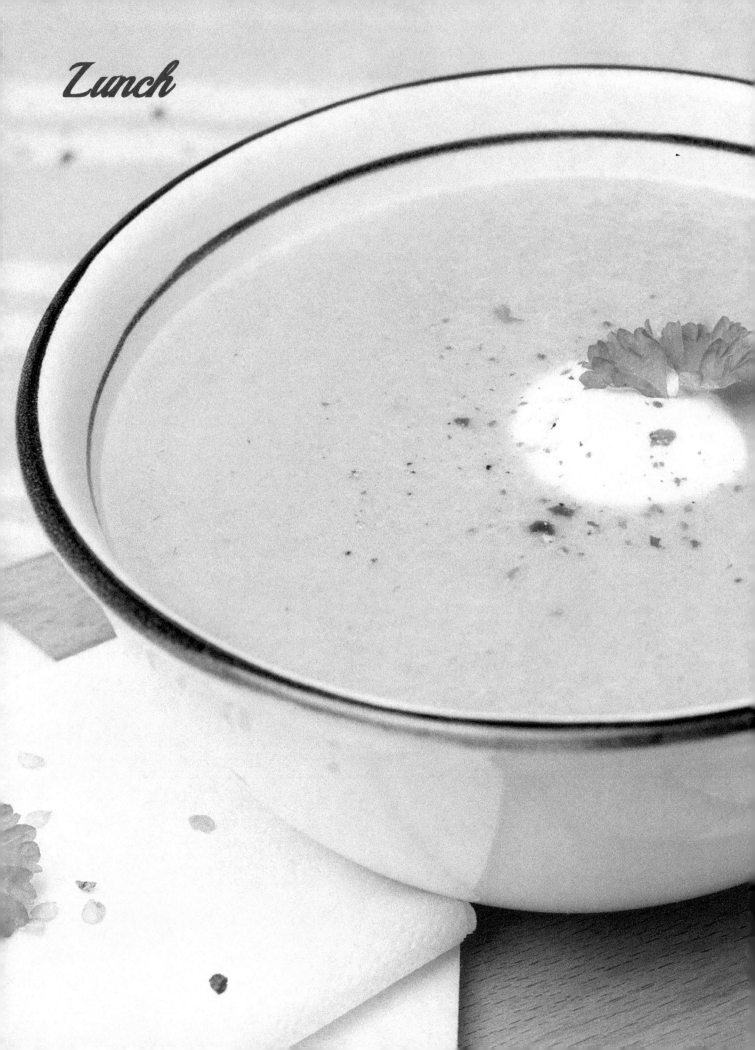
Lunch

Green Dragon Veggie Juice

Cal 73 VEGAN	Difficulty: Easy Preparation time: 5 minutes Cook time: 5 minutes Servings: 1

Nutrition per serving (g)

Fat	Saturates	Carbs	Sugars	Protein
1.1	0.2	16	5.9	4.8

Ingredients

- 1 cup ice
- ¼ large lemon
- ⅛ tsp salt
- 1 cup fresh spinach
- 1 tomato, quartered
- 2 sprigs fresh parsley
- ⅓ small jalapeño pepper
- 2 stalks celery

Method

Except for the ice and salt, add all the ingredients into a juicer and process. Stir salt in and pour juice into the cup of ice.

Tomato Juice

Cal 268
VEGAN

Difficulty: Normal
Preparation time: 60 minutes
Cook time: 25 minutes
Servings: 7

Nutrition per serving (g)

Fat	Saturates	Carbs	Sugars	Protein
3	1	58	39	13

Ingredients

- 23 lb tomatoes
- 1 cup water
- 7 tsp salt
- 3½ tsp onion salt
- 1¾ tsp celery salt

Method

1. Wash and remove the cores of the tomatoes.
2. Chop into small pieces, place in a large stockpot, and add one cup of water.
3. Set heat to medium and allow to boil.
4. Using a colander, separate the seeds and skin of the tomatoes from the juice. Discard the solid ingredients.
5. Pour juice back into the pot and allow to boil. Add salt, onion salt, and celery salt into the pot and mix.

Golden Coffee

Cal 189	Difficulty: Easy Preparation time: 2 minutes Cook time: 5 minutes Servings: 1

Nutrition per serving (g)						
Fat	Saturates	Carbs	Sugars	Fiber	Protein	Salt
8	1.5	17	10.5	5	5	0.5

Ingredients

- ½ tsp turmeric, ground
- ¼ tsp ginger, ground
- ¼ tsp cinnamon, ground
- ½ tsp black pepper, ground
- ¾ cup brewed coffee, decaffeinated
- ¼ cup coconut milk
- ½ tbsp honey

Method

1. Place the ingredients into a blender and mix well.
2. Heat through in a pot on the stove.

Vegetable Clear Soup

Cal 141
VEGAN

Difficulty: Normal
Preparation time: 10 minutes
Cook time: 40 minutes
Servings: 3

Nutrition per serving (g)

Fat	Saturates	Carbs	Sugars	Protein
2	1	22	11	5

Ingredients

- 1 large yellow onion
- 1 cup chopped celery stalks
- 1 tsp chopped ginger
- 2 cubed carrots
- 1 tsp chopped garlic
- 10 French beans
- 1½ cup mushrooms
- ½ diced cabbage
- 2 stalks celery leaves

Method

1. Into a large pot, add yellow onion, celery leaves, celery stalks, cabbage, beans, and carrots.
2. Pour water into the pot until all the veggies are immersed. Two and one-half cups of water should suffice.
3. Set your stove to low. Cover the pot and let it simmer until the veggies lose all their flavor and look wilted.
4. Using a strainer, separate the liquid from the wilted veggies.
5. Still in the strainer, mash the veggies and set aside for about 20 minutes to get even more liquid.
6. Discard the strained veggies. Into the pot containing the clear liquid, add mushrooms, ginger, and garlic. Boil until the mushrooms are soft and ready.
7. Serve.

Dinner

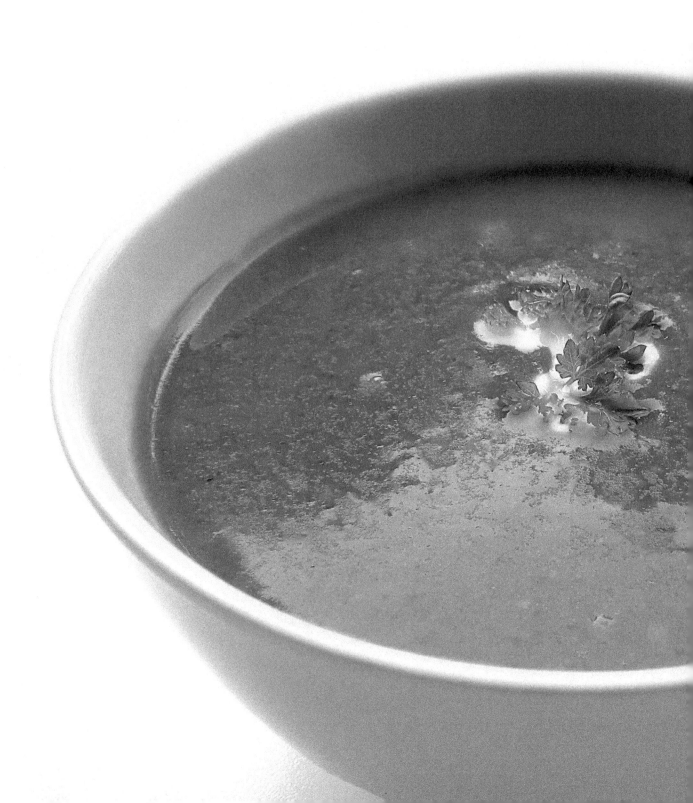

Chicken Clear Soup

Cal 172

Difficulty: Normal
Preparation time: 5 minutes
Cook time: 20 minutes
Servings: 4

Nutrition per serving (g)				
Fat	Saturates	Carbs	Sugars	Protein
11	3	2	1	14

Ingredients

- 200g boneless chicken
- ¼ tap freshly ground black pepper
- ¼ cup chopped onion
- Salt to preferred taste
- 3 smashed cloves garlic
- 4 cups water
- ¼ cup chopped carrots
- 3 sprigs thyme
- 2 bay leaves

Method

1. Wash the chicken well and place it in a pressure cooker. Add chopped onions, carrots, smashed, thyme sprigs, bay leaves, garlic cloves, and water.

2. Also, add black pepper and salt and cook on high heat for about 10 minutes. Reduce the heat to low and simmer for an additional 10 minutes. The chicken should not be overcooked, as this will prevent it from shredding right.

3. Turn off the cooler and release pressure naturally. Open the lid and separate the soup from the solid ingredients with a strainer.

4. Shred the chicken and place the pieces in four serving bowls. Pour clear soup over the chicken pieces and serve.

Japanese Clear Soup

Cal 46

Difficulty: Normal
Preparation time: 5 minutes
Cook time: 65 minutes
Servings: 10

Nutrition per serving (g)

Fat	Saturates	Carbs	Sugars	Protein
1	0	5	2	3

Ingredients

- 2 tsp sesame oil
- 10 button mushrooms, minced
- 8 cups chicken broth
- 4 whole scallions, diced
- 4 cups beef broth
- 2 inch fresh ginger, chopped
- 4 cups water
- 2 large carrots, diced
- 1 large sweet onion, chopped into wedges
- 3 smashed garlic cloves
- Salt

Method

1. Set your stove to high heat and place an 8-quart stock pot on it.
2. Heat oil in the pot and sauté carrots, onions, garlic, and ginger. The veggies should caramelize without burning.
3. Add chicken and beef broth into the pot. Also, pour in water. Boil these, then reduce the heat low. Simmer for an hour.
4. Remove the veggies from the pot with a skimmer. You may add salt to the broth now.
5. The broth can fill 10 serving bowls. Top with chopped mushrooms and scallions.

Sweet Potato Carrot Spiced Juice

Cal 318	Difficulty: Easy Preparation time: 10 minutes Cook time: 10 minutes Servings: 4

Nutrition per serving (g)				
Fat	Saturates	Carbs	Sugars	Protein
0.4	0.1	74.2	16.9	5.9

Ingredients

- ⅛ tsp ground nutmeg
- 3 large sweet potatoes, peeled
- ¼ tsp ground cinnamon
- 3 large carrots
- 1 inch fresh ginger, peeled

Method

1. Add potatoes, ginger, and carrots into a juicer and process. Add cinnamon and nutmeg into the juice and stir.

Vegan Jello

Cal 22 — VEGAN

Difficulty: Normal
Preparation time: 5 minutes
Cook time: 5 minutes
Servings: 16

Nutrition per serving (g)

Fat	Saturates	Carbs	Sugars	Protein
1	1	5	5	1

Ingredients

- 3 tbsp agar powder
- 2 cups 100% grape juice
- Olive oil cooking spray

Method

1. Prepare a 9-inch pan by coating it with cooking spray and lining it with parchment paper.
2. Thoroughly mix grape juice and agar powder in a saucepan. Then, place the pan over medium-high heat for the mixture to boil.
3. Once the agar powder has completely dissolved into the grape juice and the liquid is boiling, take the pan down.
4. Pour the grape juice mixture into the prepared pan, and place it in the refrigerator to cool. It might take two hours for the liquid to set.
5. When ready, slice the jello into small squares and serve.

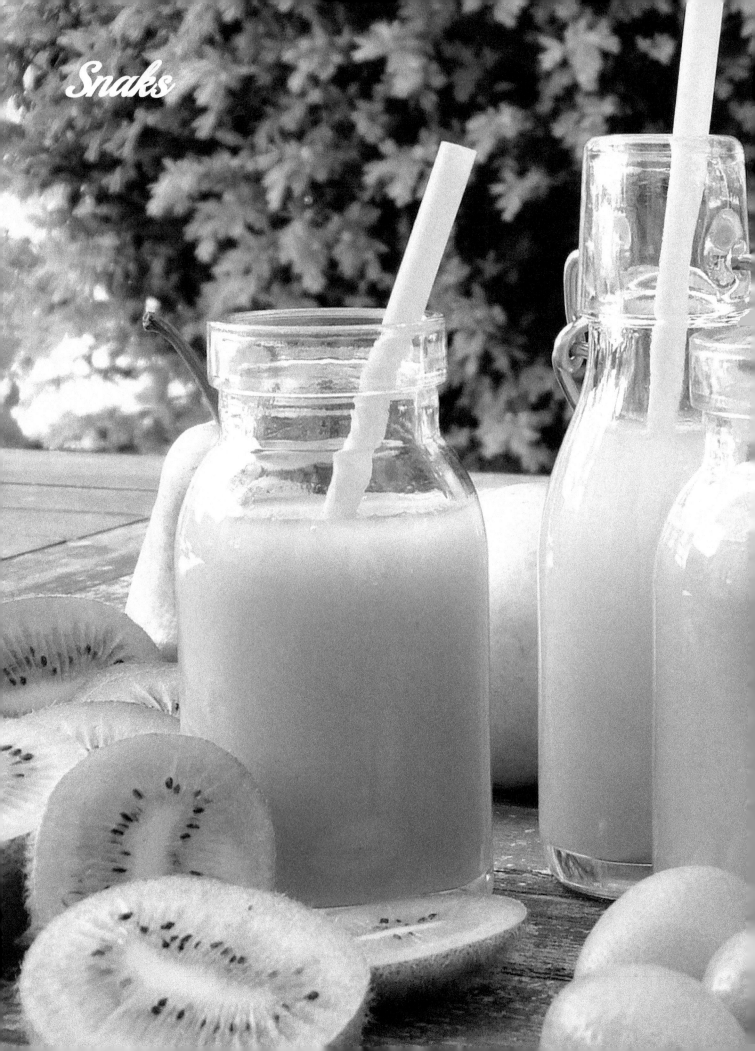

Green Smoothie Popsicles

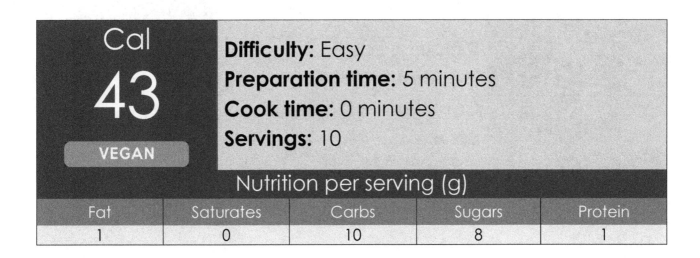

Fat	Saturates	Carbs	Sugars	Protein
1	0	10	8	1

Ingredients

- 1 cup coconut water
- 1 inch fresh ginger
- 1 cup orange juice, no pulp
- 2 cups baby spinach
- 1 ripe banana

Method

1. Peel your ginger and place it in a blender. Also, add all the ingredients into the blender and process until you get a smooth consistency.
2. Pour this mixture into a popsicle mold. Cover and leave in your freezer for about an hour.
3. Insert the wooden handles and leave for another four hours.
4. When you want to enjoy the popsicles, fill a tall bowl with warm water and dip the mold in it for about 30 seconds. When the popsicles start to loosen, gently pull the wooden handle to remove them. If the popsicles are still fixed, leave in the warm water for some more time.

Masala Chai Tea

Cal 53

VEGAN

Difficulty: Easy
Preparation time: 5 minutes
Cook time: 10 minutes
Servings: 2

Nutrition per serving (g)

Fat	Saturates	Carbs	Sugars	Protein
1	0	9	9	1

Ingredients

- ¾ cup water
- 1¼ cup dairy-free milk (like soymilk or almond milk)
- 1½ tbsp raw sugar
- 1 tsp ginger, grated (if t00 strong, use ½)
- 2 tsp loose tea
- ½ tsp Chai masala blend

Method

1. Add water, tea, ginger, masala blend, and sugar into a deep pan, and bring to a boil over medium heat. This might take up to nine minutes.
2. Stir in your dairy-free milk and allow to boil for about eight minutes.
3. Sieve to separate the solid ingredients from the liquid. Discard the solids.
4. Serve tea hot.

Strawberry Soda Syrup

Cal **306**

VEGAN

Difficulty: Easy
Preparation time: 20 minutes
Cook time: 20 minutes
Servings: 6

Nutrition per serving (g)

Fat	Saturates	Carbs	Sugars	Protein
0.5	0	78	74	1

Ingredients

- 2 cups white sugar
- 2 lb ripe strawberries, hulled and diced
- 3 cups cold water

Method

1. Set your stove to medium heat and place a saucepan on it. Add water and strawberries into the pan and bring to a boil.
2. Reduce the heat to low and simmer for about 15 minutes.
3. With a mesh strainer, separate pulp from the juice. Discard the pulp and mix sugar into the juice. Increase heat to medium and boil the juice.
4. Reduce heat to low and simmer for five minutes. Remove the foam that forms at the top of the syrup and allow it to cool.

Vegan Chai Latte

Cal 36 — VEGAN

Difficulty: Easy
Preparation time: 10 minutes
Cook time: 20 minutes
Servings: 2

Nutrition per serving (g)

Fat	Saturates	Carbs	Sugars	Protein
1.8	0.2	5	3.8	0.5

Ingredients

- 1 cup unsweetened dairy-free milk of choice (almond milk is fine)
- 1 tbsp loose leaf black tea
- Cane sugar to preferred taste
- 2 tbsp whole Chai spice blend
- 2 cups water

Method

1. Set stove to high heat and place a saucepan containing water, spice blend, and black tea on it.
2. When it starts to boil, reduce the heat to low and allow it to simmer for about 15 minutes.
3. Take the pan down and add dairy-free milk and cane sugar. Mix well and set aside for about three minutes.
4. Pour the mixture into two serving mugs and enjoy.

Watermelon Lime Agua Fresca

Cal 63
VEGAN

Difficulty: Easy
Preparation time: 15 minutes
Cook time: 60 minutes
Servings: 10

Nutrition per serving (g)

Fat	Saturates	Carbs	Sugars	Protein
0.1	0	16.4	14.8	0.5

Ingredients

- ⅓ cup lime juice, pulp-free
- 8 cups water
- ½ cup white sugar
- 5 cups watermelon, seeded and cubed

Method

1. Add watermelon, sugar, and one cup of water into a blender. Process. Transfer mixture to a pitcher and add the remaining water and lime juice. Taste to know if you should add more lime juice and sugar.
2. Keep in the refrigerator for an hour. Serve.

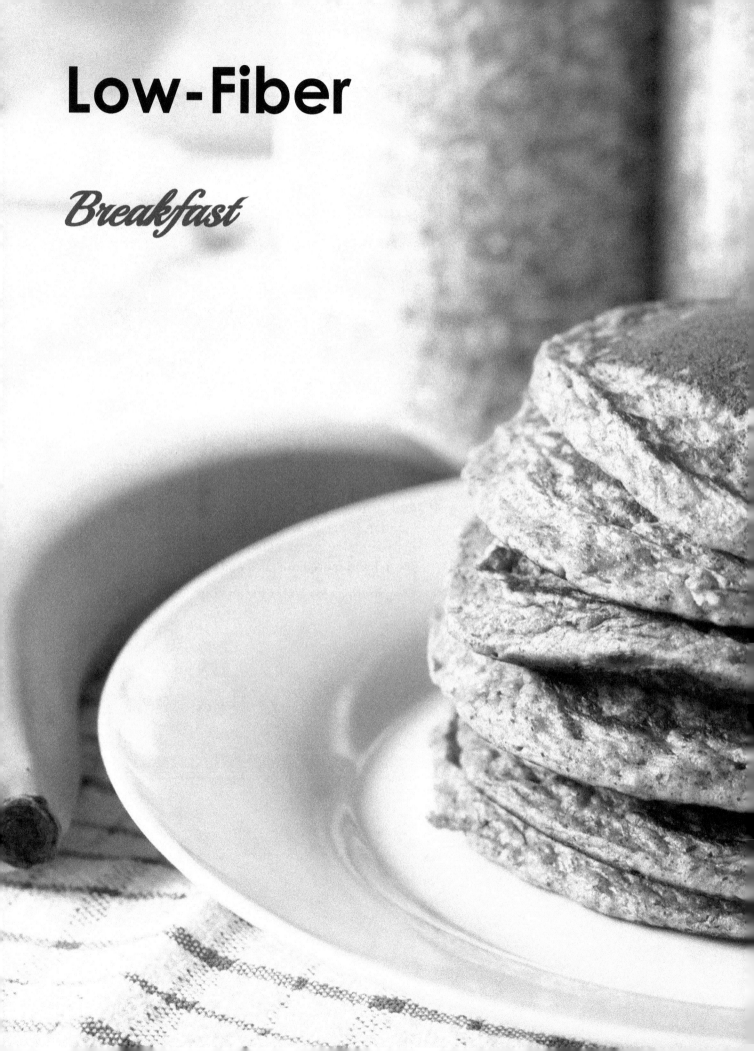

Low-Fiber

Breakfast

Almond Meal Blueberry Muffins

Cal 164	**Difficulty:** Normal **Preparation time:** 10 minutes **Cook time:** 30 minutes **Servings:** 12

Nutrition per serving (g)

Fat	Saturates	Carbs	Sugars	Protein
11.3	1.2	11.7	8.1	5.9

Ingredients

- 1 cup fresh blueberries
- 2½ ground almonds
- 1 tbsp vanilla extract
- 1¼ cups buckwheat
- 1 tsp baking powder
- 1 tsp baking soda
- 3 large fresh eggs
- ¼ cup honey
- Olive oil cooking spray

Method

1. Preheat your oven to 300 degrees F. Also, prepare a muffin pan by coating it with cooking spray.
2. Crack eggs into a bowl containing buckwheat, and whisk in honey, vanilla extract, baking powder, baking soda, and almonds. Fold the blueberries in. Transfer to the prepared pan.
3. Bake muffins in the preheated oven for about 30 minutes.
4. Allow to cool down, then serve.

Greek Yogurt Oatmeal Pancake

Cal: 161

Difficulty: Normal
Preparation time: 10 minutes
Cook time: 10 minutes
Servings: 2

Nutrition per serving (g)

Fat	Saturates	Carbs	Sugars	Protein
2.1	0.4	20.1	5	15.4

Ingredients

- ½ tsp cinnamon
- ½ cup oats
- 1 tsp sugar
- ½ cup fat-free Greek yogurt
- ½ tsp vanilla
- 4 egg whites
- ½ tsp baking powder
- Olive oil cooking spray

Method

1. Except for the oats, add all the ingredients into a blender and process until smooth. Add the oats and blend lightly. It's better if the mixture is a little chunky with oats.
2. Set your stove to medium-high heat. Grease a skillet with cooking spray and place it on the stove. Scoop the batter into the pan, ¼ cup at a time.
3. With a spatula, flip the pancakes to cook both sides.

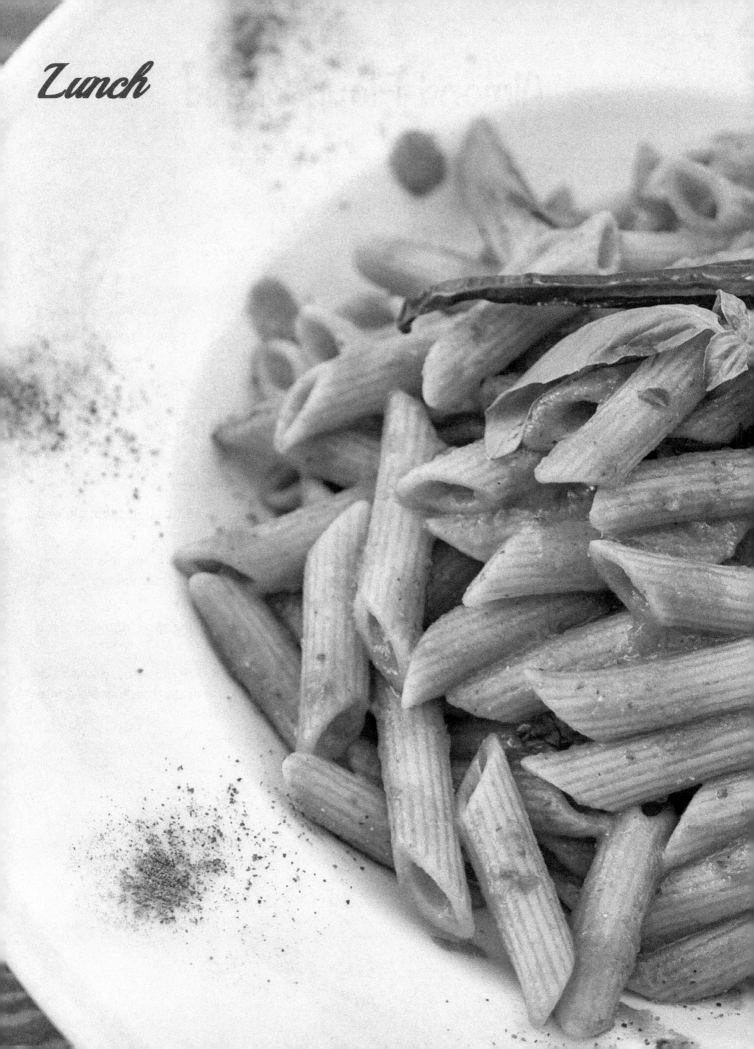

Almond Flour Bread

Cal 157

Difficulty: Normal
Preparation time: 10 minutes
Cook time: 55 minutes
Servings: 12

Nutrition per serving (g)

Fat	Saturates	Carbs	Sugars	Protein
12.9	1.2	6.6	2.3	6.6

Ingredients

- ½ tsp apple cure vinegar
- 2½ cup blanched almond flour
- ½ tsp Celtic sea salt
- 1 tbsp honey
- ½ tsp baking soda
- 3 eggs

Method

1. Preheat your oven to 300 degrees F.
2. Get a large mixing bowl and add baking soda, almond flour, and salt into it. Combine.
3. Whisk eggs in a medium sized bowl, and mix in honey and vinegar. Add the contents of the medium bowl to the dry mixture.
4. Oil a 6 by 3 loaf pan with cooking spray and scoop the egg mixture into it.
5. Place the pan in the bottom rack of the oven and bake for about 55 minutes. A knife or toothpick inserted into the bread should come out clean.
6. Allow to cool down and serve.

Chicken Fingers

Cal 45	**Difficulty:** Normal **Preparation time:** 10 minutes **Cook time:** 35 minutes **Servings:** 10

Nutrition per serving (g)

Fat	Saturates	Carbs	Sugars	Protein
0.4	0.1	5.2	0.6	5.5

Ingredients

- 1 tbsp poultry seasoning
- 1 tbsp dairy-free, gluten-free cheese (you can try Parma!)
- 8 oz chicken breast, skin and bones removed
- 1 egg
- 2 cups gluten-free corn flakes, crushed

Method

1. Make sure your oven is preheated to 400 degrees F. Also, grease a cookie sheet.
2. Slice the chicken breast into 10 strips.
3. Add poultry seasoning, corn flakes, and cheese into a bowl and mix well. Set aside.
4. Crack egg into a wide bowl. Whisk gently.
5. Dip each chicken breast strip in egg, then coat them with seasoning mix.
6. Place the strips on the prepared cookie sheet and bake for about 35 minutes.

Chicken Sour Cream Enchiladas

Cal 150

Difficulty: Normal
Preparation time: 45 minutes
Cook time: 15 minutes
Servings: 10

Nutrition per serving (g)

Fat	Saturates	Carbs	Sugars	Protein
3.3	1.3	16.3	1.1	14.2

Ingredients

- 12 oz chicken breasts
- ½ cup soy milk
- 1 cup onion, diced
- Cilantro
- Garlic powder to preferred taste
- 1 cup dairy-free cheese of choice
- Red pepper to preferred taste
- ¼ cup cashew based sour cream
- 10 corn tortillas
- ½ cup chicken soup cream

Method

1. Preheat your oven to 350 degrees F.
2. Boil the chicken to soften it. Scatter the chicken in the pot and set it aside.
3. In a saucepan, sauté onions and add it to the shredded chicken. Also, season with red pepper and garlic.
4. Warm the tortillas and set them aside.
5. Boil milk, chicken soup, and sour cream together in your saucepan.
6. Add shredded chicken to each tortilla. Top with cheese and cilantro. Drizzle with milk sauce and top with the remaining cheese.
7. Place the enchiladas in your preheated oven, and bake for 17 minutes.

Gluten-free Crustless Pizza

Cal 110

Difficulty: Normal
Preparation time: 10 minutes
Cook time: 20 minutes
Servings: 9

Nutrition per serving (g)

Fat	Saturates	Carbs	Sugars	Protein
7.9	3.5	3	1	6.8

Ingredients

- ¼ cup dairy-free cheese (Parma! is a good choice)
- 8 oz dairy-free cream cheese (soy, tofu, etc.)
- Daiya mozzarella
- 2 eggs
- ½ cup sauce
- ¼ tsp ground black pepper
- 1 tsp garlic powder

Method

1. Preheat your oven to 300 degrees F. Also, prepare a 9 by 13 baking dish by oiling it.
2. Crack eggs into a bowl and stir in dairy-free cream cheese, Parma!, garlic powder, pepper.
3. Spread the egg mixture on the baking dish and allow to bake for about 12 minutes.
4. Take the pan out and leave to cool down for 10 minutes. Add sauce to the crust and place Daiya mozzarella on top. Bake until the cheese melts. This might take up to eight minutes.

Pumpkin Muffin in a Cup

Cal 257	**Difficulty:** Easy **Preparation time:** 2 minutes **Cook time:** 1 minutes **Servings:** 4

Nutrition per serving (g)

Fat	Saturates	Carbs	Sugars	Protein
14.4	2.8	21.3	2.4	13.4

Ingredients

- 1½ tsp stevia-based sweetener
- 1 large fresh egg
- 3 tbsp canned pumpkin
- ½ tsp ground cinnamon
- ¼ ground flax
- ¼ ground nutmeg
- ½ tsp baking powder
- ½ pumpkin pie spice

Method

1. Add all the ingredients into a mug and mix well.
2. Place in the microwave for about one minute or until the muffin lightly sets.

Southern Style Cornbread

Cal 92

Difficulty: Normal
Preparation time: 10 minutes
Cook time: 20 minutes
Servings: 16

Nutrition per serving (g)

Fat	Saturates	Carbs	Sugars	Protein
0.6	0.1	20.4	6.4	2.3

Ingredients

- 2 tbsp baking powder
- 2 cup cornmeal
- ½ cup sugar
- 2 cup dairy-free milk

Method

1. Preheat your oven to 350 degree F. Also, prepare a cast iron skillet by brushing it with oil. Place the skillet in the oven to get hot.

2. Except the baking powder, mix all the ingredients in a bowl. When well combined, stir in baking powder and make sure there are no clumps.

3. Transfer the mixture to the hot skillet and bake in the oven for about 20 minutes. The cornbread should have a golden brown color by this time.

4. Divide the cornbread into 16 parts and serve.

Tomato Pasta

Cal 289 VEGAN	**Difficulty:** Normal **Preparation time:** 5 minutes **Cook time:** 20 minutes **Servings:** 8

Nutrition per serving (g)

Fat	Saturates	Carbs	Sugars	Protein
8.5	2.4	45.7	1.3	7.6

Ingredients

- 2 tbsp Extra Virgin Olive Oil
- 16 oz bag brown rice
- 6 fresh basil leaves
- ½ cup sun dried tomatoes
- Garlic powder to preferred taste
- 8 tbsp black olives, diced
- 4 oz vegan feta cheese

Method

1. Prepare the rice according to the instructions on the pack.
2. Except the oil, add every other ingredient on the list to the pot of rice. Mix well, then add olive oil. Combine properly.
3. Allow to cook for about five minutes, then serve.

Zucchini Pizza Crust

Cal 136

Difficulty: Difficult
Preparation time: 15 minutes
Cook time: 20 minutes
Servings: 2

Nutrition per serving (g)

Fat	Saturates	Carbs	Sugars	Protein
8	4.3	5	1.5	11.4

Ingredients

- 1 garlic clove, crushed
- 1 medium zucchini, grated and salted
- ½ cup dairy-free cheese, grated
- 1 egg
- Salt to taste
- Olive oil cooking spray.

Method

1. Put the zucchini in a colander and rinse it under running water. Allow it to sit in the sink for about 2 minutes to drain, then transfer to paper towels to squeeze out remaining moisture.
2. Place the zucchini in a bowl and crack your egg into it. Mix in dairy-free cheese and garlic clove.
3. Prepare an 8 by 8 pan by oiling it with nonstick spray. Spread the zucchini mixture in the pan and pat down.
4. Heat oven to 400 degrees F and bake the mixture for about 20 minutes. This should be time enough for the edges to brown.

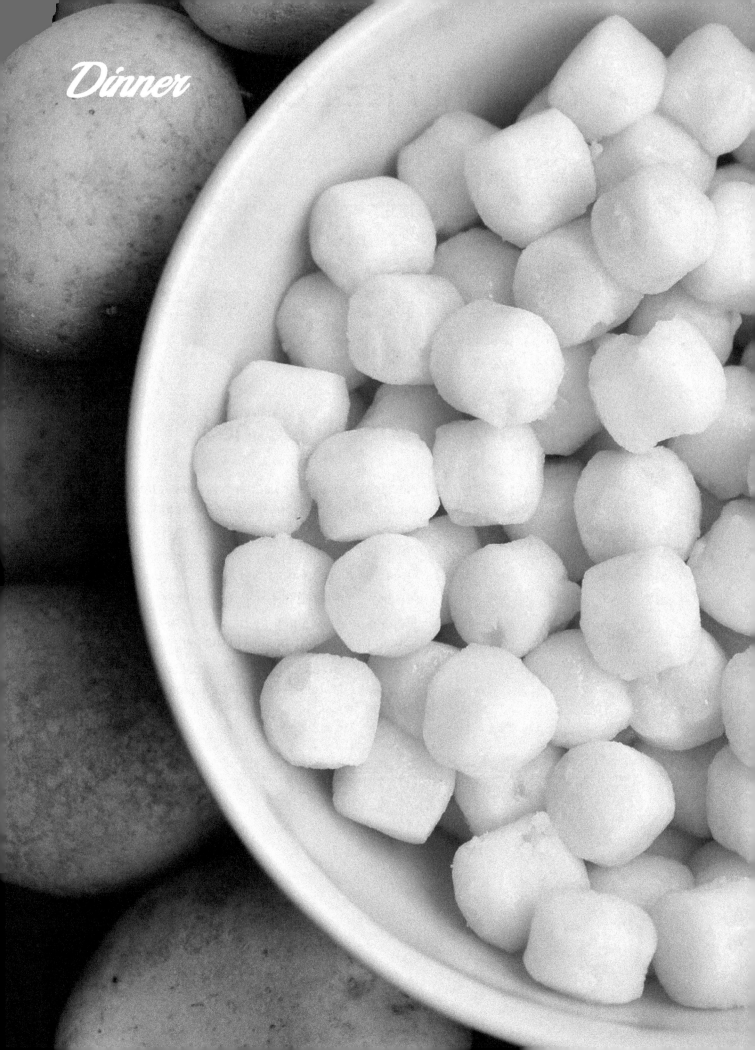

Dinner

BBQ Beef Stir-Fry

Cal 250	**Difficulty:** Normal **Preparation time:** 10 minutes **Cook time:** 20 minutes **Servings:** 6

Nutrition per serving (g)

Fat	Saturates	Carbs	Sugars	Protein
5.8	2.5	33.4	23.2	16.9

Ingredients

- 13.5 Oz bottle BBQ sauce
- 1 lb flank steak
- 1 small can bamboo shoots
- 2 large carrots
- 1 small can water chestnuts
- 2 stalk medium celery
- 2 medium scallions

Method

1. Pour some oil into a non-stick wok and place over medium heat. Cut the steak into thin strips and stir fry in the pan.
2. Add veggies into the pan and cook until they are tender. Add sauce and allow to cook.
3. This dish can be enjoyed with brown rice.

Cauliflower Rice

Cal 47

VEGAN

Difficulty: Normal
Preparation time: 20 minutes
Cook time: 20 minutes
Servings: 4

Nutrition per serving (g)

Fat	Saturates	Carbs	Sugars	Protein
0.4	0.1	10	0	3.2

Ingredients

- Olive oil cooking spray
- 1 head cauliflower, diced
- ½ cup onion, chopped
- ½ cup celery, chopped
- 1 garlic clove, chopped
- Salt to preferred taste

Method

1. Add the cauliflower into a food processor and process until the chopped veggies resemble rice.

2. Grease a large skillet with cooking spray and place it over medium heat. Add onions and celery into the pan and sauté for about 10 minutes. Next, put garlic in the pan and fry.

3. Add cauliflower, and salt to the mixture in the pan. Cover and allow to cook for 10 minutes. Stir occasionally.

Coconut Flour Bread

Cal 179	**Difficulty:** Normal **Preparation time:** 5 minutes **Cook time:** 40 minutes **Servings:** 14

Nutrition per serving (g)				
Fat	Saturates	Carbs	Sugars	Protein
18.4	14.2	1.4	0.2	3.6

Ingredients

- ½ cup melted coconut oil
- ½ cup coconut flour
- 6 eggs
- ¼ tsp Celtic sea salt
- ¼ tsp baking soda

Method

1. Make sure your oven is preheated to 350 degrees F.
2. In a bowl, mix flour, salt, and baking soda. Crack eggs one at a time into the bowl and mix well. Add oil to the mixture and combine until you get a smooth consistency.
3. Oil a bread pan with cooking spray and add the batter into the pan.
4. Allow to bake for about 40 minutes.
5. To test that the bread is ready, stick a toothpick in to see if it comes out clean. If it does, your Coconut Flour Bread is ready to be served.

90 Second Bread

Cal 166

Difficulty: Easy
Preparation time: 1 minutes
Cook time: 2 minutes
Servings: 2

Nutrition per serving (g)

Fat	Saturates	Carbs	Sugars	Protein
12.7	3.2	7.4	0.6	7.2

Ingredients

- 1 tsp coconut oil
- 1 tbsp coconut flour
- ¼ tsp baking powder
- ¼ cup almond flour
- 1 large fresh egg

Method

1. Crack your egg inside a mug and stir the other ingredients in. Combine well.
2. Microwave this mixture for about 90 seconds, then take the mug out.
3. Slide a butter knife around the side of the mug and turn it over for the bread to fall out. You should have a clean plate ready.
4. Cut the bread in two and serve.

Spaghetti Sauce With Ground Turkey

Cal 156

Difficulty: Normal
Preparation time: 10 minutes
Cook time: 20 minutes
Servings: 8

Nutrition per serving (g)

Fat	Saturates	Carbs	Sugars	Protein
7.7	1.8	11.6	6.1	13.6

Ingredients

- 2 tbsp Extra Virgin Olive Oil
- 2 cups tomato sauce, no salt added
- 4 cloves garlic
- 1 tbsp dried parsley
- 1 cup raw onions, diced
- Whole bay leaf
- 16 oz ground turkey, 93% lean
- 2 tbsp basil
- 3 tbsp ground oregano

Method

1. Set your stove to medium high heat and place a saucepan containing olive oil on it. Sauté the onion and garlic in the pan until the onions are fragrant and translucent.

2. Place the ground turkey in the pan and top with seasoning. Brown and add tomato sauce. Allow to heat.

3. You can enjoy this sauce with gluten-free spaghetti.

Sweet Potato Gnocchi

Cal 222

VEGAN

Difficulty: Difficult
Preparation time: 15 minutes
Cook time: 60 minutes
Servings: 8

Nutrition per serving (g)

Fat	Saturates	Carbs	Sugars	Protein
16.5	9.2	16	7.4	4

Ingredients

For the Brown Butter Sauce

- ½ tsp freshly ground black pepper
- ½ cup salted butter or margarine
- 2 tbsp maple syrup
- 20 fresh sage leaves
- 1 tsp ground cinnamon
- ½ tsp salt

For the Gnocchi

- 2 lb sweet potatoes
- ¼ cup hazelnuts flour
- ⅔ cup coconut milk cream cheese
- 1⅓ cup gluten-free flour
- 1½ tsp salt
- ¼ tsp freshly ground black pepper
- 1 tsp ground cinnamon

Method

To make the Gnocchi

1. Make sure your oven is preheated to 425 degrees F.
2. Insert a fork into the potatoes and let them bake for about 55 minutes. Take them out and leave to cool down.
3. Cut the potatoes into small pieces and mash them in a bowl. Add cheese, pepper, salt, and cinnamon. Mix well.
4. Slowly stir in flour until you get a soft dough. Flour a clean surface and place the dough on it. Roll into six balls and stretch each ball to long strips.
5. Place a large pot containing water over high heat. Wrap the strips around the tines of your fork and place the gnocchi in the boiling water. Repeat with the remaining gnocchi strips.
6. Cook each batch of gnocchi for about six minutes, then scoop and drain them with a slotted spoon.

To make the Brown Butter Sauce

1. With the gnocchi cooking, set another stove to medium heat and place a sauté pan on it. Melt butter in the pan and add sage leaves to the hot oil.

2. When the oil stops foaming, take the pan down and stir in the remaining sauce ingredients. Coat gnocchi with the brown butter and serve.

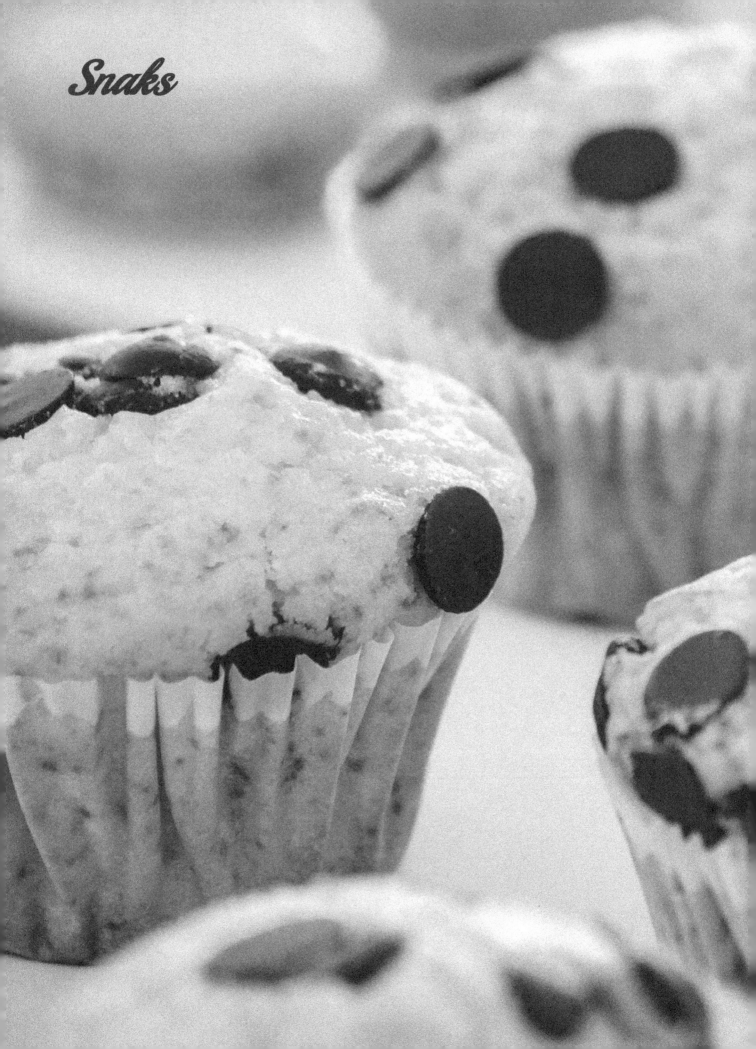

Almond and Jam Cookies

Cal 90

Difficulty: Difficult
Preparation time: 10 minutes
Cook time: 10 minutes
Servings: 20

Nutrition per serving (g)

Fat	Saturates	Carbs	Sugars	Protein
4.8	1.2	11.7	5.7	1.8

Ingredients

- 6 tbsp light butter
- 5 tsp strawberry all-fruit jam
- ½ cup granulated sugar
- ¼ tsp baking soda
- 1 egg white
- ¾ cup brown rice flour
- 1 tsp almond extract
- 1 cup almond flour

Method

1. Make sure to preheat your oven to 350 degrees F. Also, prepare a baking sheet by lining it with parchment paper.
2. Add butter to a mixing bowl and cream with a hand mixer for three minutes. Pour sugar in and mix until you get a fluffy mix.
3. Add almond extract and egg whites to the mixture and combine. Set the bowl aside.
4. In another bowl, add baking soda, rice flour, and almond flour. Mix.
5. Pour this jam mixture into the bowl containing the butter mixture. Set the hand mixer to low and combine.
6. Scoop the dough onto your prepared sheet to make 20 dough balls.
7. Press down on the balls with a spoon and add ¼ tsp jam onto each indentation.
8. Bake for 10 minutes. Allow to cool down before serving.

Almond Cookies

Cal 103

VEGAN

Difficulty: Difficult
Preparation time: 15 minutes
Cook time: 20 minutes
Servings: 12

Nutrition per serving (g)

Fat	Saturates	Carbs	Sugars	Protein
10.6	5.1	2.5	0.3	1.3

Ingredients

- 12 whole almonds
- 1 stick softened butter
- 1 tsp almond extract
- ½ cup stevia
- 1 tsp vanilla extract

Method

1. Preheat your oven to 300 degrees F. Also, prepare a cookie sheet by oiling it.
2. Into a bowl, add your softened butter. Stir in almond flour, stevia, vanilla, and almond extract. Combine well.
3. Roll this mixture into small balls and place them on the prepared sheet. You should be able to make 12 balls.
4. Bake in the oven for about five minutes before taking out the pan. Make criss-cross lines on the cookies by pressing down with a fork.
5. Place the whole almond in the center of the cookie sheet and bake for an additional 17 minutes.
6. Take the pan out of the oven, allow to cool for about five minutes, then transfer to a cooling rack.

Banana Bread

Cal 352

Difficulty: Normal
Preparation time: 10 minutes
Cook time: 30 minutes
Servings: 8

Nutrition per serving (g)

Fat	Saturates	Carbs	Sugars	Protein
3.9	0.7	57.3	20.1	4.6

Ingredients

- ¼ cup walnuts
- 2 cups white rice flour
- 1 cup stevia
- ½ cup unsweetened applesauce
- 1½ tsp baking powder
- 1½ cup mashed bananas
- ½ tsp baking soda
- 1 large egg
- ¼ tsp salt
- ¼ cup egg whites

Method

1. Make sure your oven is preheated to 350 degrees F. Also, prepare a 9 by 9 baking pan by coating it with cooking spray.
2. Put rice flour, sweetener, baking powder, baking soda, and salt into a large bowl. Combine.
3. Crack eggs into another bowl and whisk in the egg whites, mashed bananas, and applesauce. Add this to the rice flour mixture and fold.
4. Transfer the batter to your prepared pan and top with the walnuts.
5. Bake for about 30 minutes or until the bread achieves a golden brown color.
6. Take the pan out and, after the bread has cooled down, serve.

Chocolate Chip Chickpea Blondies

Cal 89

VEGAN

Difficulty: Normal
Preparation time: 12 minutes
Cook time: 25 minutes
Servings: 16

Nutrition per serving (g)

Fat	Saturates	Carbs	Sugars	Protein
5.3	1.8	10.6	7.2	1.3

Ingredients

- 1 cup vegan chocolate chips
- 15 oz can chickpeas, rinsed and drained
- ¼ tsp baking powder
- ¼ tsp baking soda
- ½ cup almond butter
- ⅓ cup agave nectar
- ½ tsp sea salt
- 2 tsp vanilla

Method

1. Dry the chickpeas and put them in a blender. Also, add ⅓ cup of chocolate chips, baking powder, soda, almond butter, salt, nectar, and vanilla into the blender. Process until you get a smooth mixture.
2. Place this mixture on an 8 by 8 pan, and top with the remaining chocolate chips.
3. Allow to bake for about 25 minutes.

Easy Peanut Butter Cookies

Cal 100

Difficulty: Easy
Preparation time: 10 minutes
Cook time: 10 minutes
Servings: 24

Nutrition per serving (g)

Fat	Saturates	Carbs	Sugars	Protein
5.5	1.1	10.7	9.3	3.5

Ingredients

- 1 egg
- 2½ cups buckwheat
- 1 tsp baking soda
- 1 tsp baking powder
- 1 cup peanut butter
- 1 cup sugar

Method

1. Preheat your oven to 350 degrees F.
2. Mix all the ingredients in a bowl and mold into 24 small balls.
3. Transfer these balls to a pan and press down with a fork to make criss-cross shape.
4. Bake in the preheated oven for 10 minutes.

Peanut Butter Brownies

Cal 220

Difficulty: Easy
Preparation time: 5 minutes
Cook time: 22 minutes
Servings: 9

Nutrition per serving (g)

Fat	Saturates	Carbs	Sugars	Protein
15.2	3.1	17.1	11.5	7.9

Ingredients

- ½ tsp baking soda
- 1 cup natural peanut butter
- 1 egg
- ½ cup honey

Method

1. Preheat your oven to 350 degrees F.
2. Using a hand mixer, combine all the ingredients until you achieve a smooth consistency.
3. Transfer this mixture to an 8 by 8 brownie pan. Allow to bake for 24 minutes.
4. Take the pan out and let the brownie cool a little for about five minutes, before placing it on a cooling rack to cool down completely.

Peanut Butter Truffle Cookies

Cal 130

Difficulty: Normal
Preparation time: 10 minutes
Cook time: 10 minutes
Servings: 24

Nutrition per serving (g)

Fat	Saturates	Carbs	Sugars	Protein
6.6	1.5	13.2	1.9	3.2

Ingredients

- ½ cup semi-sweet chocolate chips
- 2½ cup buckwheat
- 1 cup creamy peanut butter
- 1 tsp baking soda
- 1 tsp baking powder
- 1 cup brown sugar
- 1 large egg

Method

1. Preheat your oven to 350 degrees F.
2. Except for the chocolate chips, add every ingredient into a bowl and mix well.
3. When well combined, stir in the chips.
4. Get a baking sheet and scoop the dough onto the pan. Transfer to the oven and bake for about 10 minutes.
5. When the cookies are cool, serve.

Oatmeal Peanut Butter Balls

Cal 157

VEGAN

Difficulty: Easy
Preparation time: 5 minutes
Cook time: 5 minutes
Servings: 12

Nutrition per serving (g)

Fat	Saturates	Carbs	Sugars	Protein
9.4	1.3	11.9	3.5	4.6

Ingredients

- 2 tbsp honey
- ¾ cup all-natural peanut butter
- ¼ cup milled flaxseed
- 1 cup gluten-free dry rolled oats

Method

1. Add all the ingredients into a mixing bowl and mold into 12 1¼ inch balls.
2. You can eat immediately or keep in your fridge to cool.

Pumpkin Spice

Cal 199

Difficulty: Difficult
Preparation time: 10 minutes
Cook time: 7 minutes
Servings: 1

Nutrition per serving (g)

Fat	Saturates	Carbs	Sugars	Protein
5.3	0.1	18.5	6.1	21.3

Ingredients

- 13 blueberries
- ½ cup 100% pure pumpkin puree
- ⅛ salt
- 4 egg whites
- 1 tsp cinnamon
- 2 tbsp ground flaxseed meal
- 1 tsp pumpkin pie spice
- 1 tsp vanilla extract

Method

1. Add egg whites into a bowl and whisk. Stir in puree, flax meal, vanilla, salt, cinnamon, and pumpkin pie spice. Mix well.

2. Set your stove to medium heat and place a saucepan on it. Pour the mixture in your bowl into the pan, and stir while it cooks for about five minutes. By this time, the mixture should be considerably thicker.

3. Transfer Pumpkin Spice to the bowl and top with the blueberries.

Tiny Peanut Butter Cookies

Cal 55

Difficulty: Difficult
Preparation time: 15 minutes
Cook time: 9 minutes
Servings: 40

Nutrition per serving (g)

Fat	Saturates	Carbs	Sugars	Protein
3.9	0.8	3.1	2.2	2.3

Ingredients

- 1 cup natural peanut butter, unsalted
- 40 pieces semisweet chocolate chips
- ½ cup regular brown sugar
- ½ tsp vanilla extract
- ¼ cup egg substitute (like dairy-free yogurt or mashed bananas)

Method

1. Make sure your oven is preheated to 350 degrees F. Also, prepare a cookie sheet by oiling it with canola oil.
2. Add peanut butter, egg substitute, vanilla extract, and stevia into a mixing bowl and combine.
3. Scoop the dough (about a teaspoonful) into the prepared sheet. You should have up to 40 cookies. Make criss-cross lines on them with a fork.
4. Place a chocolate chip on each of the cookies and bake for about nine minutes. By this time, the bottom of the cookies should have browned.
5. Transfer the cookie sheet to a cooling rack for five minutes.

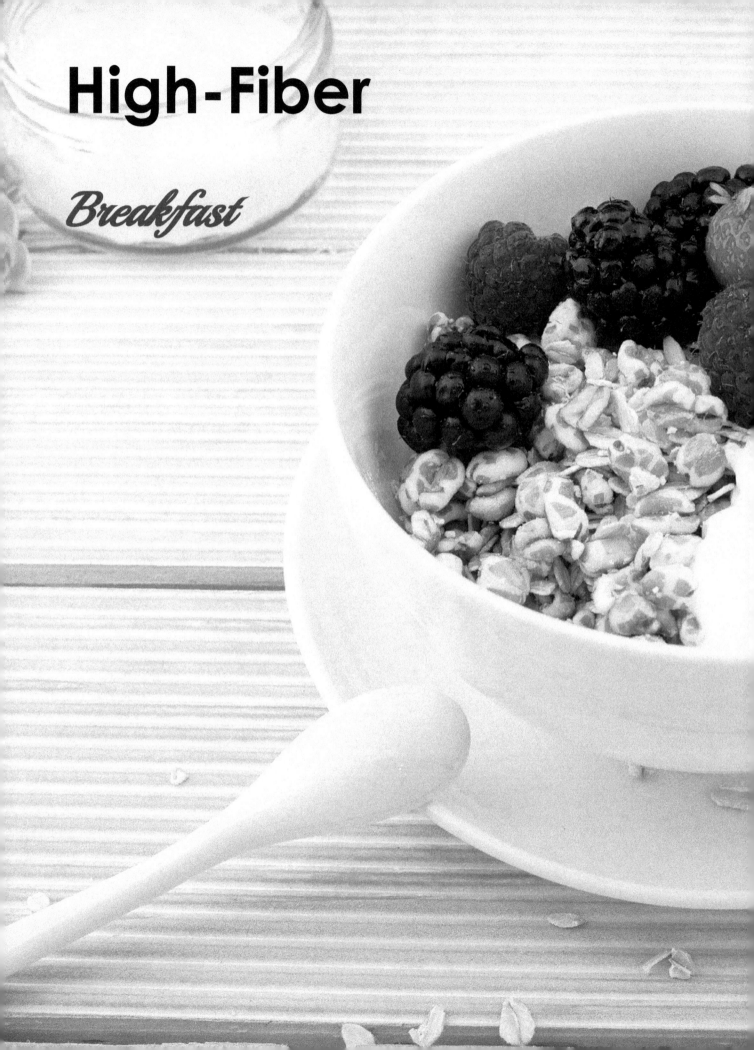

High-Fiber

Breakfast

Apple Pie Oatmeal

Cal 413	**Difficulty:** Easy **Preparation time:** 10 minutes **Cook time:** 11 minutes **Servings:** 1

Nutrition per serving (g)

Fat	Saturates	Carbs	Sugars	Protein
18	4	49	26	17

Ingredients

- 20 almonds, diced
- 1 cup soy milk
- ⅛ tsp salt
- ½ medium apple, cored and diced
- ⅛ tsp cinnamon
- ⅓ cup rolled oats
- ¼ tsp vanilla extract
- 1 tap maple syrup

Method

1. Set your stove to medium heat. Add milk and apples into a pot and place on the stove. When it begins to boil, reduce the heat to low and allow it to simmer for about five minutes. Stir while the apples and milk cooks.

2. Increase the heat to medium again, and add cinnamon, oats, salt, vanilla, and maple syrup into the pot. Stir and allow to boil. Reduce the heat to low and allow to simmer for six minutes.

3. Add almonds on top and serve.

Banana Buckwheat Pancakes and Compote

Cal 220

Difficulty: Normal
Preparation time: 13 minutes
Cook time: 20 minutes
Servings: 5

Nutrition per serving (g)

Fat	Saturates	Carbs	Sugars	Protein
4	1	38	9	9

Ingredients

- 1½ cup buckwheat
- ½ tbsp water
- 1 tsp baking soda
- 1 tsp vanilla extract (another ½ tsp to make the compote)
- 2 tsp cinnamon
- 1 tbsp coconut sugar
- 1 large banana, mashed
- 1½ cup fresh blackberries
- 2 large eggs
- ½ cup unsweetened almond milk
- Coconut oil

Method

1. Set your stove to medium-low heat and place a skillet on it.
2. While the pan heats up, mix flour, baking soda, cinnamon, mashed banana, eggs, vanilla extract, and almond milk in a bowl. Combine to form a smooth batter.
3. Oil the preheated skillet with coconut oil. Scoop ¼ cup of the cinnamon mixture into the pan and cook both sides of the pancake for two minutes each. Do the same for the remaining batter.
4. After making the pancakes, place a small saucepan over medium heat. Using a wooden spoon, mix coconut sugar, blackberries, and vanilla in the pan. Gently press down with the spoon to break the berries and stir until a thick sauce forms. If needed, add 1 tsp of tapioca starch to thick the sauce.
5. Drizzle pancake with compote, and serve.

Black Bean Spinach Quesadilla

Cal 370

Difficulty: Normal
Preparation time: 20 minutes
Cook time: 11 minutes
Servings: 4

Nutrition per serving (g)

Fat	Saturates	Carbs	Sugars	Protein
12	5	44	1	20

Ingredients

- Fresh cilantro leaves
- ½ tbsp Extra Virgin Olive Oil
- Parma
- 1 tsp chopped garlic
- 4 whole-wheat tortillas
- 8 oz cremini mushrooms, stems removed and diced
- 2 tbsp diced fresh jalapeño pepper
- ¼ tsp chili powder
- 6 oz baby spinach
- 1 cup canned black beans, rinsed and drained
- Salt to preferred taste
- Freshly ground pepper

Method

1. Set stove to medium-high heat and place a large nonstick skillet containing olive oil on it. When the oil is hot, sauté garlic in the pan for about 20 seconds. Add chili powder and mushrooms into the pan. Sauté and stir for about five minutes.
2. Add spinach, jalapeños, black beans, salt, and pepper to the mixture in the pan. Stir while they cook for three minutes. Transfer to a medium-sized bowl and clean out the pan.
3. Place tortillas on a flat, clean surface. Top with sprinkles of Parma! and add the spinach mixture on the cheese. Fold.
4. Set your stove to medium heat and place the skillet on it. Add quesadillas into the pan and cook each side for about three minutes. If more than one quesadilla can fit in the pan, add more.
5. Enjoy hot.

Chocolate Cherry Egg White Oatmeal

Cal 417

Difficulty: Normal
Preparation time: 16 minutes
Cook time: 7 minutes
Servings: 1

Nutrition per serving (g)

Fat	Saturates	Carbs	Sugars	Protein
16	1	51	17	20

Ingredients

- 1 tbsp almond butter
- ½ cup rolled oats
- ⅓ cup liquid egg whites
- ½ cup unsweetened almond milk
- ⅛ tsp salt
- ½ cup frozen cherries, thaw and diced
- ¼ tsp vanilla extract
- 1 tsp honey
- 1 tbsp unsweetened cocoa powder

Method

1. Boil a mixture of almond milk, cocoa powder, cherries, vanilla, honey, oats, and salt over medium heat. Reduce the heat to low and allow to simmer for about five minutes. Stir occasionally.
2. Take the pot down. Add egg whites into a bowl and whisk until it foams. Add oatmeal and mix well.
3. Turn the oatmeal mixture into the pot. Stir and cook on low heat for about three minutes. The oats should be considerably thicker, but do not try to hasten the process by increasing the heat. You don't want the eggs to scramble.
4. Add almond butter on top and serve.

Cinnamon French Toast

Cal 413	Difficulty: Normal Preparation time: 10 minutes Cook time: 8 minutes Servings: 1

Nutrition per serving (g)

Fat	Saturates	Carbs	Sugars	Protein
16	3	49	8	15

Ingredients

- ½ tsp vanilla extract
- 1 whole wheat tortilla
- 1 tsp cinnamon
- 1 tbsp all-natural peanut butter
- 2 eggs
- ⅓ medium banana, chopped
- 2 tbsp blueberries
- Cooking spray

Method

1. Prepare a large skillet with cooking spray and place it over medium-high heat.
2. Crack eggs into a medium-sized bowl and add vanilla and cinnamon. Whisk. Coat your tortillas entirely in the egg mixture and place flat on the skillet.
3. Cook each side of the wrap for about three minutes. Place the tortillas on a flat plate and cook the remaining egg mixture in the same pan.
4. Turn the stove off and transfer the mixture to the wraps. Also, add banana pieces, blueberries, and peanut butter.
5. Roll the tortilla and serve.

Roasted Cranberry Quinoa Oatmeal

Cal 302

Difficulty: Easy
Preparation time: 13 minutes
Cook time: 22 minutes
Servings: 3

Nutrition per serving (g)

Fat	Saturates	Carbs	Sugars	Protein
6	2	53	12	10

Ingredients

- 1 cup water
- 2 cups fresh cranberries
- 1 cup dairy-free milk
- 1 tsp coconut oil
- 1 cup gluten-free quinoa, cooked
- 1 tsp maple syrup
- 1 cup gluten-free old-fashioned oats
- ½ tsp ground cinnamon

Method

1. Make sure your oven is preheated to 425 degrees F. Also, prepare a sheet pan with parchment paper.
2. Add oil, cinnamon, maple syrup, and cranberries into the pan. Combine. Transfer the pan to the oven and bake for about 15 minutes.
3. Add water, oats, milk, and quinoa into a medium-sized pot, and allow to boil over medium heat. Stir occasionally. When the mixture starts boiling, reduce the heat to medium-low and continue cooking until the liquid reduces by half.
4. Top oatmeal with baked cranberries and serve.

Savory Cheese Oatmeal

Cal 392

Difficulty: Easy
Preparation time: 5 minutes
Cook time: 7 minutes
Servings: 1

Nutrition per serving (g)

Fat	Saturates	Carbs	Sugars	Protein
16	6	45	3	21

Ingredients

- 2 tbsp Parma
- 1 cup unsweetened almond milk
- ½ cup broccoli florets
- ⅔ cup rolled oats
- ½ cup kale leaves, diced
- ⅓ cup water
- Salt to preferred taste
- Pepper to preferred taste

Method

1. Set stove to medium-high heat and place a small pot containing water, salt, pepper, oats, almond milk, broccoli, and kale.
2. Allow this mixture to boil, then reduce heat to low and simmer for about seven minutes. Stir occasionally. The broccoli should be al dente.
3. Spread Parma! on top.

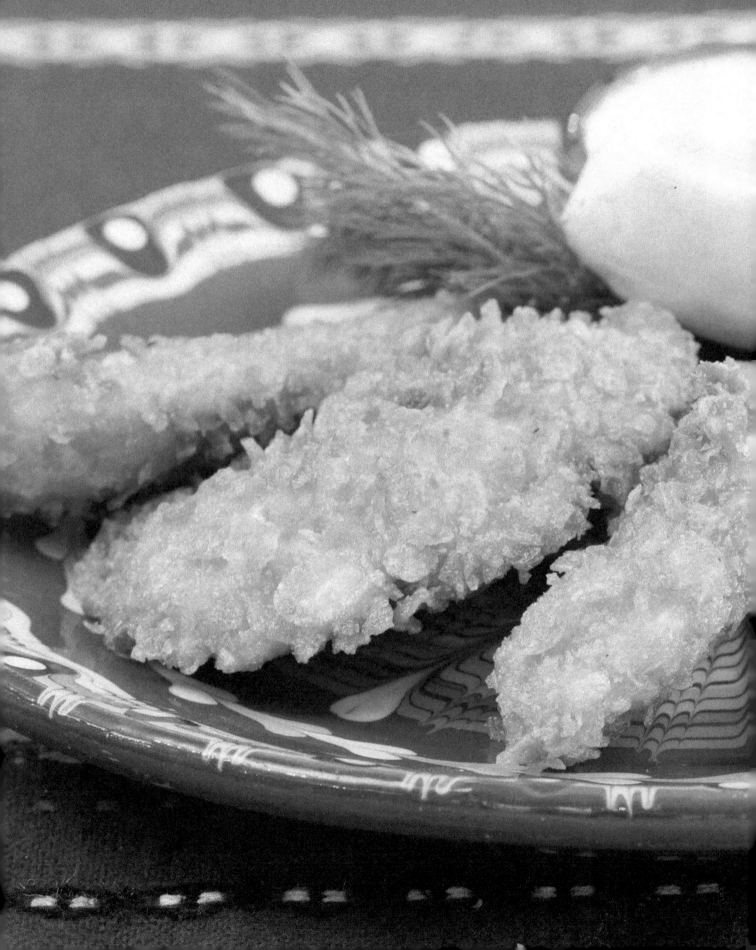

Lunch

Chicken Breast With Kabocha and Kale

Cal 533

Difficulty: Normal
Preparation time: 20 minutes
Cook time: 45 minutes
Servings: 2

Nutrition per serving (g)

Fat	Saturates	Carbs	Sugars	Protein
20	4	66	28	37

Ingredients

- 2 cups kale, diced
- 3 lb kabocha squash, peeled, halved and seeded
- ¼ tsp cumin
- 1 tbsp canola oil
- 8 oz chicken breast
- 2 tsp fresh sage, diced
- 1 tsp lemon thyme, diced
- Salt to preferred taste
- Pepper to preferred taste

Method

1. Preheat your oven to 400 degrees F.
2. Chop squash into one inch thick pieces. Into a baking sheet, mix squash, oil, sage, thyme, pepper, and salt together. Spread into a single layer.
3. Season chicken breast with salt, pepper, and cumin. Place the meat in the center of the pan.
4. Transfer the pan to the oven and bake for 35 minutes. Set the chicken aside and put kale into the baking sheet.
5. Add chicken back into the pan and cook for an additional 10 minutes. Take the pan out and remove bone from the chicken. Thinly slice the chicken breast without skinning the meat.
6. Serve.

Chicken, Parsnip, and Pomegranate Salad

Cal 540

Difficulty: Difficult
Preparation time: 20 minutes
Cook time: 27 minutes
Servings: 2

Nutrition per serving (g)

Fat	Saturates	Carbs	Sugars	Protein
21	4	65	26	27

Ingredients

- ¾ cup pomegranate seeds
- 5 medium parsnips, peeled and minced
- 6 cups arugula
- 1½ tbsp olive oil
- 2 tbsp balsamic vinegar
- ¼ tsp cumin
- 8 oz chicken breast
- Salt to preferred taste
- Pepper to preferred taste

Method

1. Preheat your oven to 450 degrees F. Also, prepare a sheet pan by lining it with parchment paper.
2. Place parsnips on the pan and pour ½ tbsp of olive oil on them. Toss and add pepper, cumin, and salt. Spread to even out the parsnip.
3. Season the chicken breast with pepper and salt, and place it in the pan. Cook in the preheated oven for about 27 minutes.
4. Set aside to cool down, then remove the bones and mince the chicken meat and skin.
5. Into a bowl, add salt, pepper, and oil. Also, add pomegranate seeds, vinegar, and arugula. Toss. Mix in the chicken and parsnips.
6. Serve.

Coconut Lentil Soup

Cal 317 — VEGAN

Difficulty: Normal
Preparation time: 15 minutes
Cook time: 45 minutes
Servings: 4

Nutrition per serving (g)

Fat	Saturates	Carbs	Sugars	Protein
6	3.1	47	4.5	21

Ingredients

- 1½ cups red lentils
- 1 tbsp curry powder
- 2½ cups water
- 1 tsp ground black pepper
- ¾ cups soy milk
- ½ red onion, diced
- ½ cup grated coconut
- 1 clove garlic, diced
- ½ inch fresh ginger, diced

Method

1. Set your stove to medium heat and place a medium saucepan over it. Add water and lentils into the pan and allow to boil.
2. Reduce the heat to low and add onions, ginger, and garlic into the pan. Simmer for about 30 minutes. By this time, the lentils should be tender.
3. Put coconut pieces and soy milk into a blender and process until you have a thick and smooth mixture. Pour this mixture over the ingredients in the pan. Mix in pepper and curry, and simmer for an additional 15 minutes.
4. Serve.

Flat-Belly Salad

Cal 390

Difficulty: Easy
Preparation time: 20 minutes
Cook time: 20 minutes
Servings: 4

Nutrition per serving (g)

Fat	Saturates	Carbs	Sugars	Protein
25	3.9	29	1.6	13

Ingredients

- 2 hard boiled eggs, grated
- 2 tbsp cider vinegar
- 1 avocado, diced
- 2 tsp whole-grain mustard
- 1 cup no-salt-added chickpeas, rinsed
- 1 tbsp shallot, thinly cut
- 14 oz can artichoke hearts, rinsed and quartered
- 8 cups mixed salad greens
- ¼ cup olive oil
- ¼ tsp pepper
- ¼ tsp salt

Method

1. In a large bowl, mix shallot, pepper, vinegar, salt, mustard, and olive oil. Add avocado, salad greens, egg shreds, artichoke, and chickpeas. Toss and serve.

Green Curry Tofu Rice

Cal 516 — VEGAN

Difficulty: Easy
Preparation time: 40 minutes
Cook time: 17 minutes
Servings: 1

Nutrition per serving (g)

Fat	Saturates	Carbs	Sugars	Protein
19	2	64	13	25

Ingredients

- 10 almonds, chopped
- 6 oz extra-firm tofu, cubed
- 2 tbsp cilantro, chopped
- 2 tbsp green curry paste
- 1 lime, zested and juiced
- 1 medium bell pepper, minced
- ¾ cup brown rice
- 3 baby radishes, minced

Method

1. Cook rice according to the directions on the pack. Set aside for later.
2. Using paper towels, squeeze out as much moisture as you can from the tofu cubes. Get a container that has a lid and put the tofu cubes and 1 tbsp of green curry paste in it. Combine and cover the container.
3. Add lime juice, lime zest, bell pepper, cooked brown rice, radishes, parsley, and the remaining curry paste into a bowl. Mix well.
4. Add the tofu and curry paste mixture in the container into the bowl. Top with chopped almonds and serve cold.

Hearty Vegetable Curry

Cal 280

Difficulty: Normal
Preparation time: 10 minutes
Cook time: 14 minutes
Servings: 4

Nutrition per serving (g)

Fat	Saturates	Carbs	Sugars	Protein
5	1	45	11	14

Ingredients

- ½ cup plain Greek yogurt
- 1½ tsp olive oil
- 2 tbsp fresh cilantro, chopped
- 1 cup sweet potato, peeled and diced
- 14½ oz can low-sodium diced tomatoes
- 1 cup small cauliflower florets
- 15 oz can chickpeas, rinsed and drained
- ¼ cup yellow onion, minced
- ¼ tsp salt
- 2 tsp curry powder
- ½ cup vegetable broth

Method

1. Set stove to medium-high heat and place a large nonstick skillet on it.
2. Sauté sweet potatoes for about three minutes, then reduce the heat to medium.
3. Add curry powder, cauliflower, and onion to the pan and cook for one minute. Stir constantly. Add salt, tomato, chickpeas, and broth into the pan and allow to boil. Reduce the heat and low and let the mixture in the pan simmer for 10 minutes. Stir occasionally.
4. Top with cilantro and enjoy with dairy-free yogurt.

Lentil Soup

Cal 348

VEGAN

Difficulty: Easy
Preparation time: 10 minutes
Cook time: 70 minutes
Servings: 6

Nutrition per serving (g)

Fat	Saturates	Carbs	Sugars	Protein
10	1.4	48	3.3	18.3

Ingredients

- 2 tbsp vinegar
- 1 onion, diced
- ½ cup spinach, rinsed, drained, and minced
- ¼ cup olive oil
- 8 cups water
- 2 carrots, chopped
- 2 cups dry lentils
- 2 stalks celery, chopped
- 14½ oz crushed tomatoes
- 1 tsp dried basil
- 2 cloves garlic, minced
- 1 bay leaf
- 1 tsp dried oregano
- Salt to preferred taste
- Ground black pepper to preferred taste

Method

1. Set your stove to medium heat and place a large soup pot containing oil on it. Cook celery, onions, and carrots in the pan for about two minutes. By this time the onions should be tender and fragrant.
2. Stir in basil, garlic, oregano, and bay leaf. Cook for another two minutes.
3. Add water lentils, and tomatoes into the pot. Allow to boil, then reduce heat and summer for an hour. Stir spinach, vinegar, salt, and pepper. Cook until the spinach wilts, and serve.

Marinated Pear and Fennel With Chickpeas

Cal 473

Difficulty: Easy
Preparation time: 20 minutes
Cook time: 0 minutes
Servings: 2

Nutrition per serving (g)

Fat	Saturates	Carbs	Sugars	Protein
23	10	52	26	20

Ingredients

- 4 oz dairy-free cheese, crumbled
- 1 medium fennel bulb, cored and diced
- ¼ cup parsley, diced
- 2 tbsp apple cider vinegar
- 15 oz can chickpeas, rinsed and drained
- 1 tbsp olive oil
- 1 medium red pear, cored and diced
- ¼ tsp salt
- ⅛ tsp paprika

Method

1. Add oil, vinegar, paprika, and salt into a container and combine. Mix in chickpeas, fennel, and pear.
2. Cover the container with a lid and leave in your refrigerator for an hour. It's better if you let it refrigerate for a day.
3. Take the container out and drain to remove excess fluid. Add parsley and cheese, and toss.

Spicy Red Lentil Soup

Cal 241
VEGAN

Difficulty: Normal
Preparation time: 15 minutes
Cook time: 30 minutes
Servings: 6

Nutrition per serving (g)

Fat	Saturates	Carbs	Sugars	Protein
1.8	0.2	41	8	16.7

Ingredients

- ½ tsp curry powder
- 1 tsp olive oil
- ½ tsp ground cayenne pepper
- 1½ cups chopped red onion
- 1 tsp ground cumin
- 28 oz can diced tomatoes
- 1½ tsp ground cardamom
- 1½ cups frozen spinach, thawed and chopped
- 2 tsp dried basil
- 2 cups dry red lentils
- 2 cups water
- Salt to preferred taste
- Pepper to preferred taste

Method

1. Place a large pot containing oil over medium heat. Cook onions in the hot oil for about two minutes, then add salt and pepper. Stir in lentils, cardamom, basil, spinach, lentils, curry powder, cumin, tomatoes, and cayenne pepper. Pour water into the pot and allow the mixture to boil.
2. Reduce the heat to low and cook for 25 minutes.
3. Carefully pour the mixture into a blender and process until smooth. Serve.

Spiced Tomato Lentil Soup

Cal 179	**Difficulty:** Normal **Preparation time:** 15 minutes **Cook time:** 20 minutes **Servings:** 5

Nutrition per serving (g)				
Fat	Saturates	Carbs	Sugars	Protein
1	0.4	32	4.2	11.1

Ingredients

- 1 tbsp Parma!
- 4 cups low-sodium vegetable broth
- 1 tbsp fresh lemon juice
- 1 small yellow onion, diced
- 14½ oz can no-added-salt tomatoes
- 1 clove garlic, diced
- 1 cup red lentils
- 1 tsp ground coriander
- Pinch cayenne pepper
- ½ tsp ground cinnamon
- Pinch garam masala
- Pinch turmeric

Method

1. Set your stove to medium-high and place a large pot containing ½ cup of vegetable broth on it. Allow to boil, then reduce heat to low.
2. Add garlic and onion into the pot and simmer for about five minutes. The onion should be soft, translucent at this point.
3. Add garam masala, coriander, cayenne pepper, turmeric, and cinnamon into the mixture in the pot. Stir and allow to simmer for about a minute.
4. Stir lentils, remaining broth, and tomatoes into the pot. Increase the heat to medium-high and allow the mixture to boil. Then, reduce the heat to low and simmer for about 12 minutes.
5. Take the pot down and pour lemon juice into the soup. Stir and serve. Garnish with sprinkles of Parma!

Sweet Potato Chili

Cal 507 — VEGAN

Difficulty: Difficult
Preparation time: 15 minutes
Cook time: 6 hours
Servings: 4

Nutrition per serving (g)

Fat	Saturates	Carbs	Sugars	Protein
20	5	59	11	27

Ingredients

- 1 medium avocado, diced
- 2 tbsp olive oil
- ¼ cup fresh parsley, chopped roughly
- 1 medium yellow onion, diced
- ¼ cup fresh basil, chopped roughly
- 5 garlic cloves, diced
- 4 cups low-sodium chicken stock
- 2 tbsp tomato paste
- 15 oz kidney beans, rinsed and drained
- 1 tbsp chili powder
- 15 oz canned tomatoes
- 8 oz lean ground beef
- 4 medium sweet potatoes, chopped into 1 inch cubes
- Salt & Pepper

Method

1. Set stove to medium heat and place a large skillet containing olive oil on it. Sauté the onions for about three minutes and add in garlic. Cook for one minute and add chili powder and tomato paste. Stir while this mixture cooks for a minute.

2. Raise the heat to medium-high and add beef. Add salt and pepper, and brown the beef. This should take three minutes. Remember to stir while it cooks.

3. Add chicken stock, tomatoes, beans, potatoes, salt, and pepper to the mixture in the pan. Stir well. Reduce the heat to low and cook for about six hours.

4. Garnish with chopped parsley, avocado, and basil.

Sweet Potato Salad

Cal 531

Difficulty: Easy
Preparation time: 10 minutes
Cook time: 6 minutes
Servings: 2

Nutrition per serving (g)

Fat	Saturates	Carbs	Sugars	Protein
20	7	67	14	21

Ingredients

- 2 oz dairy-free cheese, crumbled
- 2 medium-sized sweet potatoes
- 1 large cucumber, seedless and cut into 1 inch bits
- ½ medium-sized ripe avocado
- 1½ cups black beans, rinsed and drained
- ¼ cup plain low-fat Greek yogurt
- ¼ tsp paprika
- 1 lime, zested and juiced
- 2 tsp olive oil
- Salt to preferred taste
- Pepper to preferred taste

Method

1. Gently stab all around the potatoes with a fork. Cover them with wet paper towels, set your microwave to high, and cook the potatoes for about six minutes. By this time, they should be soft. Allow to cool and chop them into one inch bits.

2. Add yogurt, avocado, olive oil, paprika, lime zest, lime juice, salt, and pepper into a food processor and blend until you get a smooth mixture.

3. Add black beans, scallions, cucumber, and cooked potatoes into a bowl. Pour the yogurt dressing on top and combine.

4. If you like, top with cheese. Serve.

Swiss Chard Wraps With Chicken

Cal 500

Difficulty: Difficult
Preparation time: 15 minutes
Cook time: 30 minutes
Servings: 2

Nutrition per serving (g)

Fat	Saturates	Carbs	Sugars	Protein
20	4	53	10	31

Ingredients

- 1 lime, juiced
- 2 medium-sized sweet potatoes, cubed
- 1 tsp tahini
- 1 tsp olive oil
- ½ medium-sized avocado, diced
- ¼ tsp paprika
- 1 cup chickpeas, rinsed and drained
- Salt to preferred taste
- Pepper to preferred taste
- 4 Swiss chard leaves, remove stems
- 8 oz chicken breast, season with salt and pepper

Method

1. Preheat your oven to 450 degrees F. Also, prepare a sheet pan by lining it with parchment paper.
2. Add oil and potatoes into the pan. Toss and season with pepper, salt, and paprika. Spread for an even layer.
3. Place seasoned chicken in the pan and bake for about 25 minutes. A thermometer placed in the center of the chicken should read 165 degrees F. Allow the chicken to cool down before removing the bone and mincing the meat.
4. Set stove to medium heat and place a saucepan containing three inches of water on it. Add salt and allow to boil. Set the saucepan down and pour cold water into a bowl.
5. Dip Swiss chard into the pan of hot water for about 15 seconds, then transfer to the bowl of cold water. Dry with paper towels.
6. Add lime juice, chickpeas, tahini, and diced avocados into a bowl. Mash this mixture.
7. Spread ¼ avocado mixture on a chard leaf. Add ¼ chicken pieces and potatoes on top and wrap the leaf tightly. Repeat with the remaining Swiss chard leaves. Enjoy.

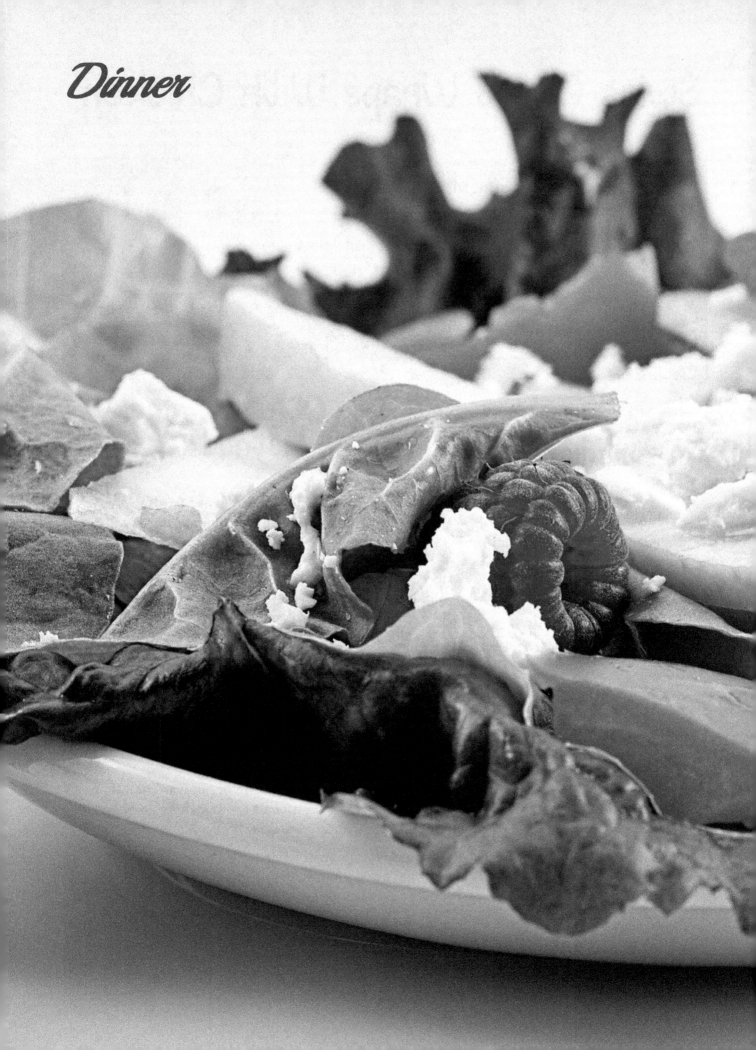

Dinner

Baked Potato With Ground Beef and Broccoli

Cal 537

Difficulty: Difficult
Preparation time: 10 minutes
Cook time: 60 minutes
Servings: 1

Nutrition per serving (g)

Fat	Saturates	Carbs	Sugars	Protein
18	6	64	15	31

Ingredients

- 2 cups broccoli florets, chopped
- 1 medium russet potato
- 2 tsp soy sauce
- 1 tsp olive oil
- 1 tsp Dijon mustard
- 1 small yellow onion, diced
- 2 tbsp tomato paste
- 3 oz lean ground beef
- ¼ cup low-sodium chicken stock
- ¼ tsp paprika
- Salt to preferred taste
- Pepper to Preferred taste

Method

1. Preheat your oven to 425 degrees F.
2. Wash the potato and season it with salt and pepper. Place on a sheet tray and bake for 50 minutes.
3. Set your stove to medium heat and place a skillet containing oil on it. Add onions, salt, and pepper into the pan and stir while it cooks for about five minutes.
4. Add paprika and ground beef into the pan and continue cooking for another two minutes. Stir occasionally and scatter the beef.
5. Reduce the heat to low and pour in the stock. Also, add mustard, tomato paste, and soy sauce. Stir well.
6. Add the broccoli and cook for an additional five minutes. By the time, the mixture should be thick and the broccoli, al dente (cooked, but not too soft).
7. Cut the baked potato horizontally and place on a flat plate. Add beef mixture inside the potato.

Broccoli Cheddar Brown Rice

Cal 543

Difficulty: Normal
Preparation time: 15 minutes
Cook time: 22 minutes
Servings: 1

Nutrition per serving (g)

Fat	Saturates	Carbs	Sugars	Protein
22	8	60	5	25

Ingredients

- 1 oz dairy-free cheese, crumbled
- 2 tsp canola oil
- ⅛ tsp curry powder
- ½ small yellow onion, thinly cut
- ¼ tsp paprika
- 2 garlic cloves, diced
- 2 tbsp nutritional yeast flakes
- 1½ cups broccoli florets
- 2 tbsp plain Greek yogurt, 2 percent fat
- 1 cup brown rice, cooked
- 1 tbsp water
- Salt to preferred taste
- Pepper to preferred taste

Method

1. Preheat your oven to 400 degrees F.
2. Set your stove to medium heat and place a cast iron skillet containing 1 tsp oil on it. When it heats up, cook onions in the pan for about two minutes. Then, add garlic, salt, and pepper and cook for an additional minute.
3. Reduce the heat to medium-low and add water broccoli. Stir while it cooks for about two minutes. Add the rice and continue stirring for another two minutes. Take the pan down and turn off the heat.
4. Add yogurt, curry powder, yeast flakes, paprika, and the remaining oil into a bowl and mix. Add this mixture to the ingredients in the pan and combine. Spread to even out and add cheese on top.
5. Transfer the pan to the preheated oven and bake for about 15 minutes. The cheese should have browned by this time.
6. Allow to cool, then serve.

Brussels Sprouts and Sweet Potato Hash

Cal 529

Difficulty: Normal
Preparation time: 12 minutes
Cook time: 34 minutes
Servings: 1

Nutrition per serving (g)

Fat	Saturates	Carbs	Sugars	Protein
20	4	64	10	29

Ingredients

- 1 large egg
- 1 medium sweet potato, minced
- 2 tbsp fresh basil leaves, diced
- 10 Brussels sprouts, halved
- ⅔ cup canned black beans, rinsed and drained
- 2 tsp canola oil
- ¼ tsp chili powder
- Salt to preferred taste
- Pepper to preferred taste

Method

1. Preheat your oven to 400 degrees F.
2. Mix Brussels sprouts, chili powder, pepper, potato, oil, and salt in an oven-safe skillet. Transfer to your oven to bake for about 30 minutes. The potato should be tender by this time.
3. Take the skillet out and allow it to cool down for about three minutes. Set your stove to medium heat and place the pan on it. Stir in basil and beans, and crack your egg into the pan. Cook for about four minutes. The yolk should remain runny, but the white should set.

Flank Steak Tacos

Cal 531

Difficulty: Difficult
Preparation time: 20 minutes
Cook time: 10 minutes
Servings: 1

Nutrition per serving (g)

Fat	Saturates	Carbs	Sugars	Protein
22	5	55	3	33

Ingredients

- ¼ medium ripe avocado, minced
- 4 oz flank steak, trim off fat
- 3 small corn tortillas
- 1 lime, juiced and zested
- ½ tbsp fresh basil leaves
- ¼ tsp chili powder
- ½ medium beefsteak tomato, seeded and diced
- 2 tsp canola oil
- 4 cherries, pitted and diced
- ¼ canned black beans, rinsed and drained
- Salt to preferred taste
- Pepper to preferred taste

Method

1. Get a sealable container and add a pinch of chili powder, 1 tsp oil, ½ lime juice, salt, pepper, and steak in it. Shake well to coat the steak and leave in a refrigerator for a day or an hour.
2. Add the remaining juice, another pinch of chili powder, lime zest, basil, beans, tomato, cherries, salt, and pepper into a bowl. Mix well and keep in the refrigerator.
3. Take the container out of the refrigerator, dry the steak, and set it aside. Throw the marinade away.
4. Set your stove to medium-high heat and place an oven-safe skillet on it. Add the remaining oil and let it heat up.
5. Cook the steak in the oil for six minutes. That is, three minutes for both sides of the steak. If the oil gets too hot and starts to smoke, reduce to medium.
6. Remove the steak from the pan and allow it to cool down for about five minutes. Cut into three thin slices.
7. Wipe oil from the skillet and, over medium heat, cook tortillas for one minute.
8. Take the bean salsa from the refrigerator and serve on top of the tortillas. Also, top with avocado and steak.

Greek Chicken Pasta

Cal 487

Difficulty: Normal
Preparation time: 15 minutes
Cook time: 15 minutes
Servings: 6

Nutrition per serving (g)

Fat	Saturates	Carbs	Sugars	Protein
11	2.8	70	5	32.6

Ingredients

- 2 tsp dried oregano
- 16 oz pack linguine pasta
- 2 tbsp lemon juice
- ½ cup chopped red onion
- 3 tbsp chopped fresh parsley
- 1 tbsp olive oil
- ½ cup Parma!
- 2 cloves garlic, crushed
- 1 large tomato, diced
- 1 lb skinless and boneless chicken breast, minced
- 14 oz can marinated artichoke hearts, rinsed, drained, and diced
- 2 lemons, cut into wedges
- Salt to preferred taste
- Pepper to preferred taste

Method

1. Set your stove to medium-high heat and place a pot of salted water on it. Cook paste in the pot according to the direction on the pack.

2. When the pasta is ready, place a skillet containing oil on the stove. Sauté garlic and onion in the pan for about two minutes, then add the diced chicken breasts. Cook for about 6 m9, until the chicken loses its pink color. Stir occasionally.

3. Reduce the heat to medium-low and stir lemon juice, parsley, artichoke hearts, oregano, tomatoes, Parma!, and the cooked pasta into the pan.

4. Stir and cook for three minutes. Take the pan down and season Greek Chicken Pasta with salt and pepper. Top with lemons.

Grilled Zucchini Hummus

Cal 332 — VEGAN

Difficulty: Normal
Preparation time: 15 minutes
Cook time: 6 minutes
Servings: 2

Nutrition per serving (g)

Fat	Saturates	Carbs	Sugars	Protein
17	6	34	2	13

Ingredients

- 4 tbsp hummus
- 1 medium zucchini, thinly cut vertically
- 2 large tortillas
- 1 slice dairy-free cheese
- 1 tbsp Extra Virgin Olive Oil
- 1 cup kale, stem removed
- 1 medium-sized tomato
- ⅛ cup red onion, chopped
- Salt to preferred taste
- Pepper to preferred taste

Method

1. Set your stove to medium heat and place a skillet on it.
2. In a bowl, add oil, salt, and pepper. Add the zucchini slices and toss. Cook all the sides of zucchini in the skillet for five minutes.
3. Remove the zucchini from the pan and replace with tortillas. Cook for one minute.
4. Spread tortilla wraps on a flat plate and arrange 2 tbsp hummus, tomatoes, one slice dairy-free cheese, onion, zucchini, and ½ cup kale into each one.
5. Roll tightly and serve.

Parmesan Cauliflower With Chickpeas

Cal 525

Difficulty: Normal
Preparation time: 15 minutes
Cook time: 35 minutes
Servings: 1

Nutrition per serving (g)

Fat	Saturates	Carbs	Sugars	Protein
23	5	64	22	23

Ingredients

- ½ oz dairy-free cheese, grated
- ⅓ large cauliflower, chopped to fill 3 cups
- 1 tbsp fresh basil, diced
- 1 cup chickpeas, rinsed and drained
- ⅓ cup pomegranate seeds
- 1 tbsp olive oil
- ¼ tsp cumin
- 1 tsp fresh sage, chopped
- Salt to preferred taste
- Pepper to preferred taste

Method

1. Preheat your oven to 400 degrees F. Prepare a baking sheet by lining it with parchment paper.
2. Add oil, cauliflower florets, sage, chickpeas, and cumin into the sheet pan, and toss. Add salt and pepper, and combine well. Spread the ingredients to get an even layer, and transfer the pan to the oven.
3. Bake for about 35 minutes, then take the pan out. Add grated dairy-free cheese of choice, pomegranate seeds, and basil. Combine and serve.

Rainbow Veggie Chili

Cal 187 — VEGAN

Difficulty: Normal
Preparation time: 20 minutes
Cook time: 75 minutes
Servings: 8

Nutrition per serving (g)

Fat	Saturates	Carbs	Sugars	Protein
5	0.7	34	5.8	7.4

Ingredients

- ¼ tsp cayenne pepper
- 2 tbsp olive oil
- ½ tsp ground black pepper
- 1 zucchini, minced
- ½ tsp ground oregano
- 1 yellow squash, minced
- 1 tbsp chili powder
- 1 red bell pepper, chopped
- 28 oz can crushed tomatoes
- 15 oz can chili beans in spicy sauce
- 4 cloves garlic, minced
- 1 green bell pepper, chopped
- 6 oz can tomato paste
- 1 onion, diced
- 1 fresh jalapeño pepper, diced

Method

1. Set your stove to medium-high heat and place a large pot containing olive oil on it. Add squash, bell peppers, zucchini, onion, jalapeño, and garlic into the pot. Allow to cook for about five minutes.

2. Add crushed tomatoes with the marinade, chili beans in spicy sauce, tomato paste, corn, and black beans into the pot. Combine. Stir in cayenne pepper, chili powder, black pepper, and oregano. Allow to boil, then reduce the heat to low and simmer for about an hour.

3. Serve.

Roasted Pork Loin With Apple Jus

Cal 506	**Difficulty:** Normal **Preparation time:** 20 minutes **Cook time:** 42 minutes **Servings:** 3

Nutrition per serving (g)

Fat	Saturates	Carbs	Sugars	Protein
18	2	64	23	28

Ingredients

- 5 cups kale leaves, stemmed and minced
- 4 medium-sized sweet potatoes, cubed
- 1 large apple, cored and diced
- 3 tbsp canola oil
- 1 tbsp honey
- ¼ tsp cumin
- 1 cup low-sodium chicken stock
- 8 oz boneless pork loin, center cut
- 8 garlic cloves, diced
- Salt to preferred taste
- Pepper to preferred taste

Method

1. Preheat your oven to 400 degrees F. Also, prepare a sheet pan by lining the insides with parchment paper.
2. Pour 1 tbsp of oil into the pan and add sweet potatoes. Toss and season with pepper and salt. Dry the pork loin and season with pepper and salt.
3. Set your stove to medium-high heat and place a skillet containing 1 tbsp of oil. Cook pork loin in the pan for about four minutes. That is, two minutes for each side. The pork should be lightly browned.
4. Take the pork from the pan and place on the baking sheet with the potatoes. Reserve the liquids in the skillet.
5. Cook for about 20 minutes or until the potatoes are tender. Take the baking sheet out and when the pork has cooled down a bit (about five minutes), thinly slice it.
6. Place the skillet containing pork juices over medium heat. Cook garlic in the pan for a minute. Stir occasionally.

7. To make the jus, add chicken stock, chopped apples, and honey into the skillet and cook for about 20 minutes. The liquid should reduce and the apples should be tender.

8. Transfer the jus to a bowl and clean out the pan. Place the pan over medium heat and add the remaining oil. When it heats up, add kale, salt, and pepper. Cook for about five minutes. Stir occasionally.

9. Serve pork, potatoes, and kale on flat plates. Drizzle with the jus.

Salmon Quinoa and Roasted Brussel Sprouts

Cal 537

Difficulty: Normal
Preparation time: 10 minutes
Cook time: 10 minutes
Servings: 1

Nutrition per serving (g)

Fat	Saturates	Carbs	Sugars	Protein
24	3	54	4	30

Ingredients

- 1 tbsp fresh parsley, diced
- 5 Brussels sprouts, minced
- ½ medium avocado, chopped into ½ inch cubes
- 1 tsp olive oil
- 1 tsp rice vinegar, unseasoned
- 3 oz salmon, skinned and filleted
- ⅔ cup quinoa, cooked
- Salt to preferred taste
- Pepper to preferred taste

Method

1. Preheat your oven to 450 degrees F.
2. Add oil, Brussels sprouts, salt, pepper into an oven-safe skillet. Toss and spread evenly.
3. Season the skinned salmon and place in the skillet. Transfer the pan to the oven and cook for seven minutes. Thicker fillets might require more time.
4. Add vinegar, quinoa, parsley, Brussels sprouts, and avocado into a bowl and mix. Place salmon on this mixture and serve.

Sheet Pan Salmon

Cal 530	**Difficulty:** Normal **Preparation time:** 10 minutes **Cook time:** 10 minutes **Servings:** 1

Nutrition per serving (g)

Fat	Saturates	Carbs	Sugars	Protein
19	2	65	17	28

Ingredients

- 3 oz salmon gullet, skinned
- 1 cup kale leaves, diced
- ¼ tsp cumin
- 1 medium apple, cored and diced
- ⅛ tsp salt (extra to season salmon)
- 1 cup quinoa, cooked
- ⅛ tsp pepper (extra to season salmon)
- 2 tsp canola oil

Method

1. Preheat your oven to 450 degrees F. Also, line a baking sheet with parchment paper.
2. Add oil, kale, cumin, quinoa, apples, salt, and pepper to the pan. Toss. Season the salmon fillets with salt and pepper, and add to the pan.
3. For medium-rare, cook salmon in the preheated oven for 10 minutes. For well done, cook salmon for 10 minutes, discard the kale mixture, and cook salmon for another five minutes.

Spicy Black Bean Burgers

Cal 343

Difficulty: Normal
Preparation time: 30 minutes
Cook time: 14 minutes
Servings: 4

Nutrition per serving (g)

Fat	Saturates	Carbs	Sugars	Protein
13	2	41	3	11

Ingredients

For the Black Bean Burgers

- 4 whole-wheat potato rolls
- 15 oz can reduced-sodium black beans, rinsed and drained
- ¼ tsp kosher salt
- ½ red bell pepper, diced
- 1 tbsp ground cumin
- ½ cup scallions, diced
- 1 tsp cayenne pepper hot sauce
- 3 tbsp fresh cilantro, diced
- 1 large egg
- ½ cup quick cooking oats
- 3 cloves garlic
- Olive oil cooking spray

For the Chipotle Mayo topping

- 1 tbsp Chipotle chili in adobo sauce, diced
- 3½ tbsp mayonnaise

Method

To make the Black Bean Burgers

4. Prepare a baking sheet by lining it with wax paper.
5. Pat the beans dry and put in a medium-sized bowl. Using a fork, mash the beans until it forms a paste.
6. Add bell pepper, garlic, scallions, and cilantro into a food processor and blend well. Also, blend oats, cumin, egg, hot sauce, and salt. Place this mixture on the bean paste and fold.
7. Wet or oil your hands, then mold the paste into four patties. Place the patties on the prepared baking sheet, and transfer to your refrigerator. If the patties are too moist, you can 1 tbsp of oats. Freeze for two hours.
8. Set your stove to medium heat and place a nonstick skillet on it. Oil the pan with cooking spray and cook the patties until browned. Cook both sides for seven minutes each.
9. Cover the burgers with buns.

To make the Chipotle Mayo

10. Mix chili and mayo in a bowl. Pour over the burgers.

Superfast Asparagus

Cal 530

VEGAN

Difficulty: Easy
Preparation time: 5 minutes
Cook time: 10 minutes
Servings: 3

Nutrition per serving (g)

Fat	Saturates	Carbs	Sugars	Protein
19	2	65	17	28

Ingredients

- 1 tsp Cajun seasoning
- 1 lb asparagus
- Olive oil cooking spray

Method

1. Preheat your oven to 425 degrees F.
2. Break the asparagus at the soft part and place the spears on a sheet pan. Spread into an even layer. Oil with cooking spray and top with Cajun seasoning.
3. Bake in the oven for about 10 minutes. Serve.

Sweet Potato With White Bean Bake

Cal 537

VEGAN

Difficulty: Normal
Preparation time: 10 minutes
Cook time: 55 minutes
Servings: 2

Nutrition per serving (g)

Fat	Saturates	Carbs	Sugars	Protein
22	10	59	10	28

Ingredients

- ⅔ cup white beans, rinsed, drained, and mashed
- ½ cup low-sodium vegetable stock
- 4 Swiss chard leaves, diced
- 2 oz soy-based cheese
- 2 medium-sized sweet potatoes, cut into 1½ inch pieces
- 2 tbsp nutritional yeast flakes
- 1 tbsp olive oil
- 1 tsp fresh sage, diced

Method

1. Preheat your oven to 400 degrees F.
2. Set your stove to medium heat and place a large skillet containing a mixture of olive oil, stock, cheese, sage, and yeast on it.
3. Stir while it cooks until you get sauce. Add Swiss chard, potatoes, and beans into the pan and toss. Even them out and transfer the pan to your oven to bake for about 45 minutes.
4. Take the pan out when the potatoes are well done. Serve after they have cooled down.

Wilted Kale, Chickpeas, and Quinoa

Cal 596

VEGAN

Difficulty: Normal
Preparation time: 13 minutes
Cook time: 35 minutes
Servings: 2

Nutrition per serving (g)

Fat	Saturates	Carbs	Sugars	Protein
19	2	68	10	23

Ingredients

- 1 lemon, juiced
- 15 oz chickpeas, rinsed and drained
- 2 tbsp nutritional yeast flakes
- 2 tsp olive oil
- 2 tbsp tahini
- ¼ tsp paprika
- 1 cup quinoa, cooked
- 4 cup kale leaves, diced
- Salt to preferred taste
- Pepper to preferred taste

Method

1. Preheat your oven to 400 degrees F. Also, line a baking sheet with parchment paper.
2. Add chickpeas to the pan and pour oil over them. Sprinkle salt, paprika, and pepper on top and mix.
3. Place the baking sheet in the oven and bake for 25 minutes. Take the pan out and mix in kale. Return to the oven and bake for another 10 minutes.
4. Add quinoa to the baked chickpeas and toss.
5. Mix lemon juice, tahini, and yeast flakes in a bowl. Pour this sauce over the chickpea mixture and serve.

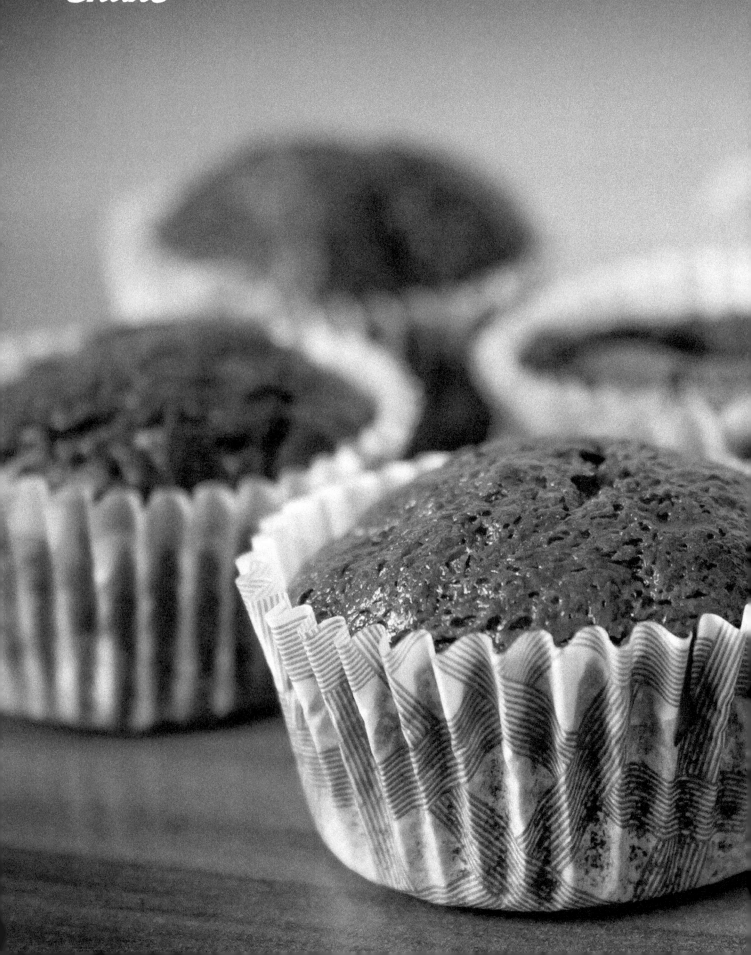

Banana Nuts Overnight Oats

Cal 428

Difficulty: Easy
Preparation time: 15 minutes
Cook time: 0 minutes
Servings: 1

Nutrition per serving (g)

Fat	Saturates	Carbs	Sugars	Protein
19	3	49	12	19

Ingredients

- 7½ pecans, chopped
- ½ large ripe bananas, mashed
- ¼ tsp cinnamon
- ½ cup rolled oats
- ¼ tsp vanilla extract
- ½ cup plain 2 percent Greek yogurt
- ⅓ cup unsweetened almond milk

Method

1. Except for the pecans, add every ingredient on the list into a small, sealable bowl and combine.
2. Cover the bowl and refrigerate for about six hours.
3. Top with pecans and enjoy cold.

Kale and Pear Smoothie

Cal 228

Difficulty: Easy
Preparation time: 10 minutes
Cook time: 0 minutes
Servings: 1

Nutrition per serving (g)

Fat	Saturates	Carbs	Sugars	Protein
22	0	56	26	6

Ingredients

- ¾ cup cold water
- 2 cups raw kale
- ¼ cup ice
- 1 large pear, cored and diced
- ½ lemon, juiced
- ½ cucumber, peeled

Method

1. Add all the listed ingredients into a blender, and process until you get a smooth mixture. Feel free to add more water if the smoothie is too thick.

Yogurt With Pumpkin Granola

Cal 389	**Difficulty:** Easy **Preparation time:** 10 minutes **Cook time:** 40 minutes **Servings:** 2			
	Nutrition per serving (g)			
Fat	Saturates	Carbs	Sugars	Protein
17	3	46	20	17

Ingredients

- 1 cup 2 percent fat Greek yogurt
- ¾ cup rolled oats
- 3 tbsp raisins
- ¼ cup canned pumpkins
- 7½ pecans, diced
- 1 tbsp olive oil
- ¼ tsp pumpkin pie spice
- 1 tbsp maple syrup

Method

1. Preheat your oven to 300 degrees F. Also, line a baking sheet with parchment paper.
2. Add oats, pumpkin pie, oil, canned pumpkin, chopped pecans, and syrup into a bowl and mix.
3. Scoop the oats mixture onto the prepared pan and spread. Bake for 40 minutes. Toss halfway through. Spread raisins on top of the granola and combine.
4. Add Greek yogurt into a serving bowl and top with the granola.

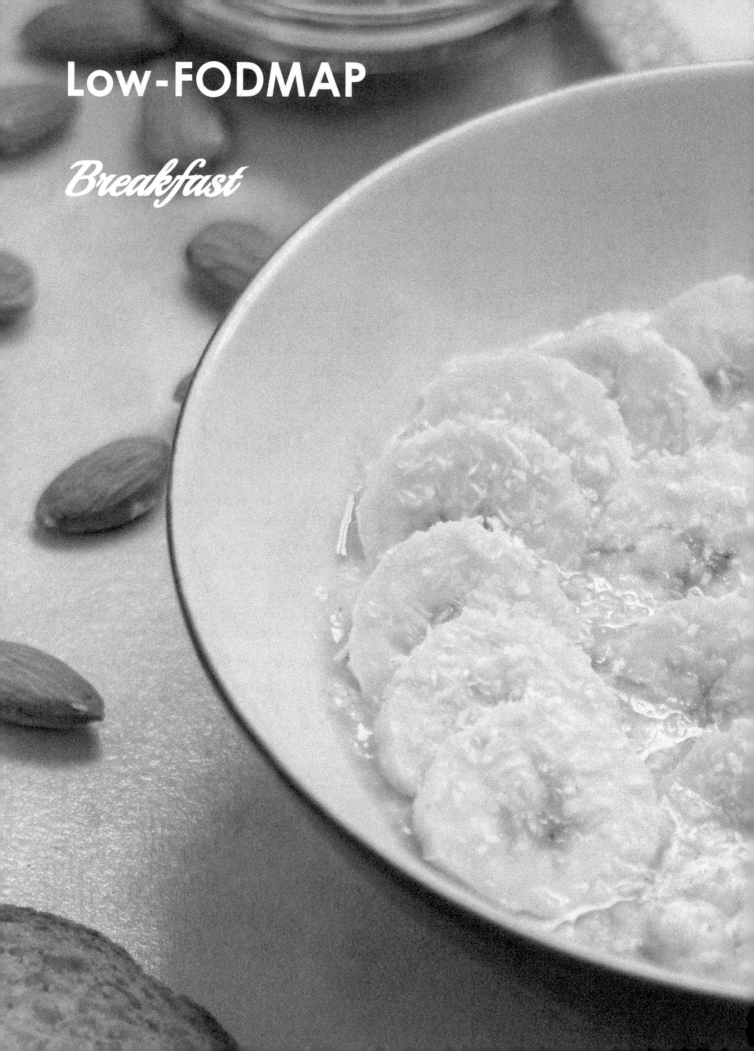

Low-FODMAP

Breakfast

Egg Wraps

Cal 414

Difficulty: Easy
Preparation time: 5 minutes
Cook time: 5 minutes
Servings: 4

Nutrition per serving (g)

Fat	Saturates	Carbs	Sugars	Fiber	Protein	Salt
33	8	2	2	0	25	0.2

Ingredients

- Oil to grease the pan (from the approved food list: avocado, olive, or sunflower)
- 4-8 eggs
- Pinch of salt
- Pepper

Method

1. Grease a non-stick pan with oil then place over medium heat to warm.
2. Whisk the egg in a bowl and pour it into the pan, ensuring it is spread evenly. Add in salt and pepper to taste.
3. Cook for 30-60 seconds on each side; gently flip when the edges on the first side are cooked.
4. Place on a plate to cool and repeat with the remainder of the eggs.

Tip

When using a small or medium pan (6-8 inches), cook one egg at a time. If using a large pan (10-12 inches), cook 2 eggs at a time.

Banana Porridge

Cal 450
VEGAN

Difficulty: Easy
Preparation time: 2 minutes
Cook time: 5 minutes
Servings: 1

Nutrition per serving (g)

Fat	Saturates	Carbs	Sugars	Fiber	Protein	Salt
14.7	1.4	73.3	25.4	7.6	7.8	0.2

Ingredients

- ½ cup rolled oats
- ½ cup almond milk
- ⅓ cup banana, sliced
- 2 tsp sunflower oil
- 2 tsp maple syrup
- ¼ tsp vanilla extract
- Pinch of cinnamon

Method

1. Cook the oats according to the instructions and use almond milk.

2. Combine oil, syrup, cinnamon, and vanilla in a saucepan over medium heat. Let the mixture bubble for a minute and add the banana. Cook for 3 minutes. The banana should look plump.

3. Serve the oats with the banana on top.

Banana Oatcakes

Cal 530	**Difficulty:** Easy **Preparation time:** 34 minutes **Cook time:** 32 minutes **Servings:** 4

Nutrition per serving (g)

Fat	Saturates	Carbs	Sugars	Fiber	Protein	Salt
12.5	2.75	80	5.5	14.5	21.25	0.2

Ingredients

- 1 unripe banana
- 1 egg
- ½ cup rice milk
- 1 tbsp Greek yogurt
- 1 ½ cups rolled oats
- ⅓ cup oat flour
- 2 tsp cinnamon
- Pinch of salt

Method

1. Mash the banana in a bowl and add the egg, milk, and yogurt, whisking after each ingredient. Next, add the dry ingredients, making sure to mix thoroughly.

2. Let the mixture rest for 15-30 minutes.

3. Grease a pan with low-FODMAP-approved oil and place it on medium heat.

4. Pour ¼ of the batter into the pan and flip when it begins bubbling. Remove the oatcake when it is golden brown on both sides.

5. Repeat 3 more times until you have 4 oatcakes.

6. Add a low-FODMAP-approved topping if desired.

Pineapple, Strawberry, Raspberry Smoothie

Cal 110
VEGAN

Difficulty: Easy
Preparation time: 2 minutes
Cook time: 3 minutes
Servings: 2

Nutrition per serving (g)

Fat	Saturates	Carbs	Sugars	Fiber	Protein	Salt
2.5	0	23	12.5	5	2	0.2

Ingredients

- 1 banana, frozen and sliced
- ½ cup strawberries, fresh or frozen
- ¼ cup pineapple, fresh
- ½ cup raspberries, frozen
- 1 cup almond milk, can substitute other approved milk

Method

Place ingredients in a blender and blend. Add more milk to create a thinner consistency.

Blueberry, Lime, and Coconut Smoothie

Cal 186 — VEGAN

Difficulty: Easy
Preparation time: 2 minutes
Cook time: 5 minutes
Servings: 2

Nutrition per serving (g)

Fat	Saturates	Carbs	Sugars	Fiber	Protein	Salt
13.5	5	14	8.5	3	4.5	0.2

Ingredients

- ½ cup blueberries, fresh or frozen
- 2 tbsp coconut flakes
- 2 tbsp lime juice
- ⅔ cup FODMAP-approved yogurt or vegan yogurt
- 1 tsp chia seeds
- 2 tbsp water
- Ice, when using fresh blueberries (Approximately 6 cubes, depending on the desired texture)

Method

Blend all ingredients together until frothy.

Crepes and Berries

Cal 277

Difficulty: Easy
Preparation time: 18 minutes
Cook time: 8 minutes
Servings: 4

Nutrition per serving (g)

Fat	Saturates	Carbs	Sugars	Fiber	Protein	Salt
10.5	4.5	25	6	3.5	8	0.2

Ingredients

Crepes

- ½ cup oat flour
- 1 tsp brown sugar
- 1 tsp white sugar
- 2 eggs
- 1 ½ tbsp melted butter
- 1 tsp vanilla extract

Filling

- ½ cup berry mix
- Pinch of brown sugar
- Pinch of cinnamon
- 2 tbsp Greek yogurt

Method

1. In a blender, place the crepe ingredients and blend for two minutes. Set aside to rest for 15 minutes.

2. Mix the brown sugar and cinnamon with the berries.

3. After the crepe mix has rested, place a non-stick pan, greased with oil, over medium heat. Add ¼ cup of the crepe batter to the pan. Gently move the pan to cover the bottom of the pan with a thin layer of batter. Cook for a minute and gently flip.

4. Once the crepes are cooked, place them on a plate and top with a small amount of yogurt, fold, and place the berries on top.

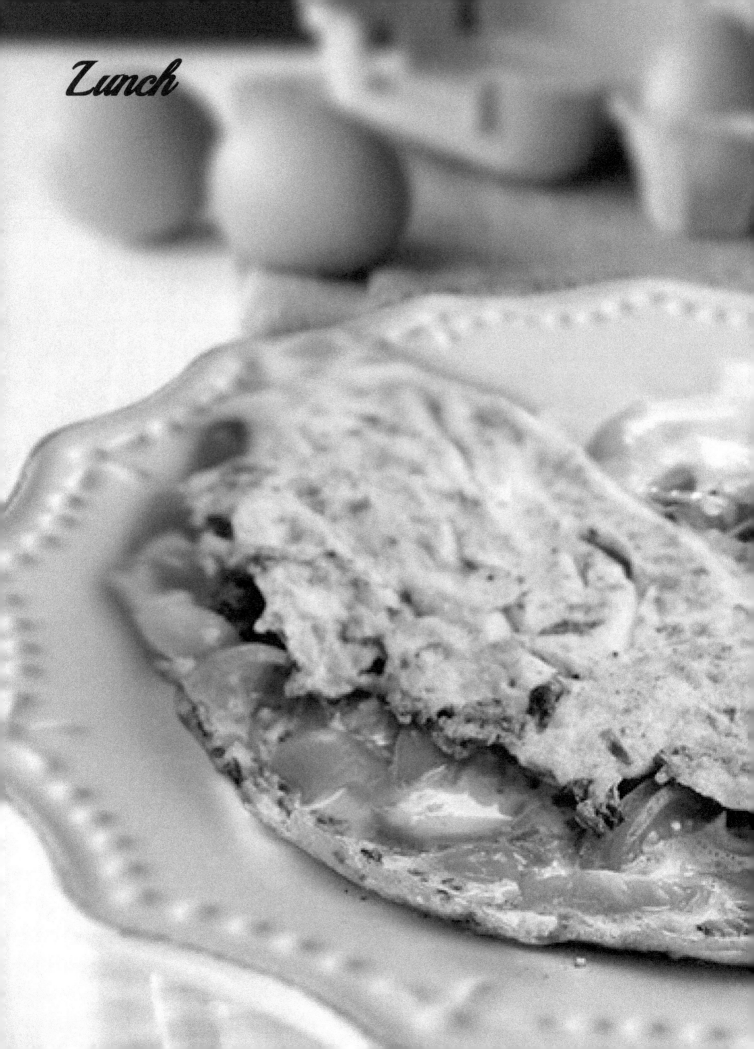

Tomato and Green Bean Salad

Cal 125

Difficulty: Easy
Preparation time: 3 minutes
Cook time: 5 minutes
Servings: 6

Nutrition per serving (g)

Fat	Saturates	Carbs	Sugars	Fiber	Protein	Salt
8.8	2	10.8	4.5	1.8	2.5	0.5

Ingredients

- 1 cup green beans
- ½ cup mayonnaise
- ½ cup Greek yogurt
- 1 tbsp chopped basil
- 2 tbsp chopped parsley
- Pinch of salt
- Pinch of pepper
- 2 tbsp lactose-free or another FODMAP-approved milk
- 1 tbsp Dijon mustard
- 2 tomatoes
- 2 spring onions, green part only
- 1 ½ cups lettuce

Method

1. In a bowl, mix mayonnaise, yogurt, milk, mustard, basil, parsley, salt, and pepper.

2. Wash the green beans, lettuce, and spring onions, then drain the water and chop the green onions. Shred the lettuce into a separate bowl and mix in the green beans and spring onions.

3. Cut the tomatoes into quarters and mix into the bowl. Put the dressing into a serving jug and serve.

Corn Salad

Cal 189 — VEGAN

Difficulty: Easy
Preparation time: 2 minutes
Cook time: 5 minutes
Servings: 2

Nutrition per serving (g)

Fat	Saturates	Carbs	Sugars	Fiber	Protein	Salt
8	1.5	17	10.5	5	5	0.5

Ingredients

- 1 can (15 oz) corn
- 1 cup cherry tomatoes
- 1 cup cucumber
- 2 spring onions, green parts only
- 1 red capsicum
- 2 tbsp mayonnaise (vegan)

Method

1. Slice the tomatoes in half.
2. Cut the cucumber into slices and then quarters. Chop the green part of the spring onion finely.
3. Thinly slice the capsicum.
4. Mix all the ingredients with the mayonnaise in a bowl and serve.

Pesto Noodles

Cal 569

Difficulty: Easy
Preparation time: 5 minutes
Cook time: 10 minutes
Servings: 2

Nutrition per serving (g)

Fat	Saturates	Carbs	Sugars	Fiber	Protein	Salt
50	5.5	26	1.5	3	6	0.2

Ingredients

Pesto

- ¾ cup basil, fresh
- 2 tbsp garlic-infused oil
- ¼ cup pine nuts
- 2 tbsp olive oil
- Pinch of salt
- Pinch of pepper
- ½ cup Parmesan, grated

Noodles

- 1 cup rice noodles

Method

1. In a food processor, mix basil, garlic oil, and pine nuts until coarsely chopped.

2. Add the olive oil, cheese, salt, and pepper to the processor and mix until the pesto is fully mixed and smooth.

3. Cook the noodles according to the instructions on the packet. Once cooked, toss the noodles in a bowl with 3 tablespoons pesto and mix until the noodles are covered.

4. Serve!

Chicken Wrap

Cal 392

Difficulty: Easy
Preparation time: 5 minutes
Cook time: 0 minutes
Servings: 4

Nutrition per serving (g)

Fat	Saturates	Carbs	Sugars	Fiber	Protein	Salt
12.7	4.7	17.7	3.5	5.5	22.7	0.2

Ingredients

- 1 ½ cups chicken, cooked and chopped
- 3 cups lettuce, chopped
- 20 cherry tomatoes, halved
- ¼ cup Parmesan, grated
- Pinch of pepper
- 4 gluten-free wraps, can substitute with other low-FODMAP-approved wraps

Method

1. In a bowl, mix together all the ingredients, leaving the wraps to the side.

2. Lay the wraps out and place ¼ of the mixture onto the center. Roll up. If taking to eat on the go, use a toothpick to secure the wrap.

Quiche in Ham Cups

Cal 190

Difficulty: Easy
Preparation time: 10 minutes
Cook time: 20 minutes
Servings: 6

Nutrition per serving (g)

Fat	Saturates	Carbs	Sugars	Fiber	Protein	Salt
8.5	5.1	11.8	1.6	1.6	9.5	0.3

Ingredients

- 6 slices ham, cold cut, rounded
- 1 small bell pepper, diced
- ½ cup spring onion, green tips only
- 4 eggs, beaten
- 2 tbsp rice flour
- 4 tbsp lactose-free milk, can be substituted with other approved milk
- Pinch of salt
- Pinch of pepper

Method

1. Preheat the oven to 350°F and line 6 muffin tins with the ham slices.
2. Mix together the flour and milk, whisking constantly.
3. Add in the eggs, salt, and pepper, mixing until smooth. Add the spring onion and bell pepper. Pour carefully into the ham cups.
4. Bake for 15-20 minutes. It's ready when the quiche is puffy and the ham is crispy.
5. Let cool for 10 minutes then use a knife to carefully lift the quiche out of the tins.

Feta, Chicken, and Pepper Sandwich

Cal 601

Difficulty: Easy
Preparation time: 5 minutes
Cook time: 20 minutes
Servings: 2

Nutrition per serving (g)

Fat	Saturates	Carbs	Sugars	Fiber	Protein	Salt
27	12.5	40	4	6	46	0.3

Ingredients

- 1 chicken breast fillet
- 1 tsp olive oil
- 4 slices gluten-free or spelt sourdough bread
- 1 cup feta cheese
- 1 large red capsicum, deseeded and cut into strips
- ¼ cup basil

Method

1. Cut the chicken in half to create thin fillets, drizzle olive oil over them, and season with salt and pepper. Place into a frying pan that has been heated over medium heat. Cook the fillets for 3 minutes on each side. Remove and cover with foil for 5 minutes before cutting into strips

2. Drizzle some oil onto one side of each slice of bread.

3. Assemble the sandwich by placing the feta, chicken, pepper, and basil, divided onto two slices of bread with the oil side down. Top with the other two slices of bread with the oil side facing up.

4. Cook the sandwiches in a frying pan for 3 minutes on each side until the bread is golden.

5. Remove from heat and serve.

Rice & Zucchini Slice

Cal 201	**Difficulty:** Medium **Preparation time:** 5 minutes **Cook time:** 55 minutes **Servings:** 4

Nutrition per serving (g)

Fat	Saturates	Carbs	Sugars	Fiber	Protein	Salt
14	9.8	7.8	3.5	2	11.9	0.3

Ingredients

- ⅔ cup rice (brown, white, or basmati)
- ⅔ cup water
- 1 cup grated zucchini
- ½ cup grated carrot
- 3 eggs, beaten lightly
- 1 cup grated cheddar cheese

Method

1. Preheat the oven to 350°F. Line the base and sides of a loaf pan with parchment paper, leaving space for overhang.

2. Add rice and water to a saucepan and cook according to instructions on the packet.

3. In a bowl, add the zucchini, eggs, ½ cup cheese, rice, and carrot and mix well. Spread evenly over the bottom of the pan. Spread the remainder of the cheese over the top.

4. Bake for 30-35 minutes. When it's finished, the top should appear golden. Let cool before cutting into quarters. Place into a microwaveable, airtight Tupperware and put into the fridge within 2 hours of baking.

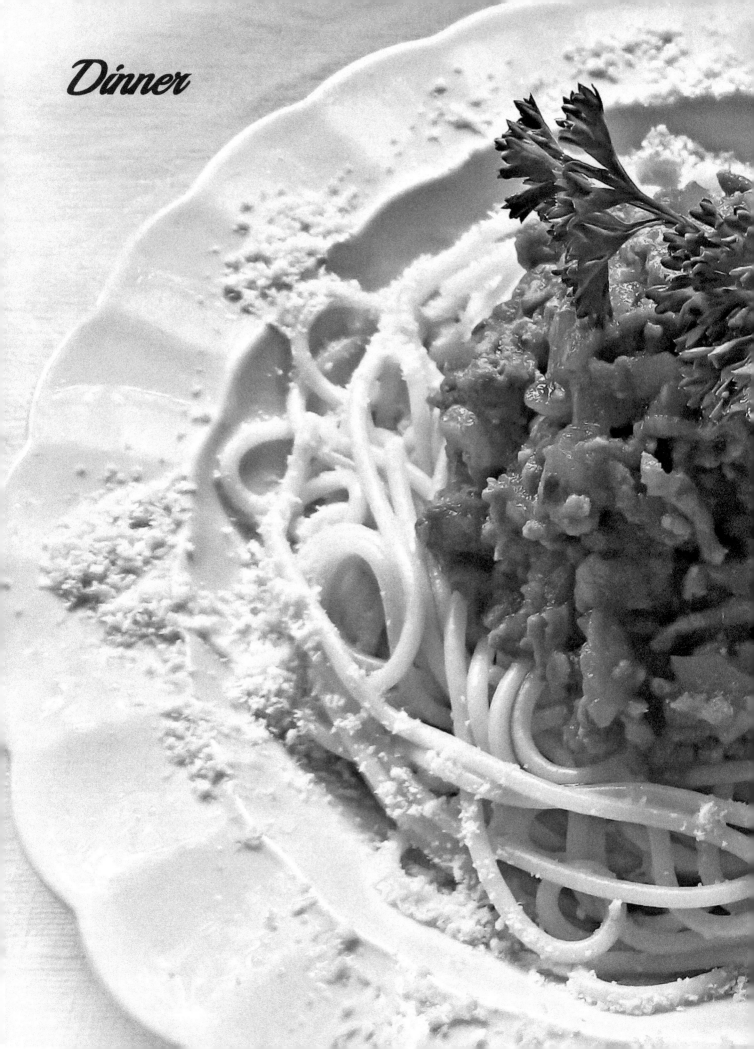

Dinner

Bolognese

Cal 642

Difficulty: Normal
Preparation time: 5 minutes
Cook time: 40 minutes
Servings: 4

Nutrition per serving (g)

Fat	Saturates	Carbs	Sugars	Fiber	Protein	Salt
19	7.3	39.7	11	14.7	39.7	0.5

Ingredients

- 1 tbsp olive oil
- 1 lb ground beef, lean
- ½ cup leeks, tips only
- 1 can (14 oz) tomatoes, crushed
- 3 tbsp tomato paste
- 1 tsp oregano, dried
- 1 tsp thyme, dried
- 4 cups baby spinach
- Pinch of salt
- Pinch of pepper
- 1 ½ cups gluten-free spaghetti
- ½ cup approved cheese, grated
- 2 large carrots, peeled and cut into sticks
- ⅔ cup green beans

Method

1. Chop the spinach and leeks. Peel the carrots and cut into sticks. Slice the green beans. Put to one side.

2. Place a large pan over medium heat with olive oil in it. Cook the ground beef until it is browned. Add the tomatoes, leeks, spinach, and herbs to the beef. Mix well and let simmer for 20 minutes. Stir occasionally to ensure it does not burn. Season to taste.

3. In a large pot, add water and a generous amount of salt. Bring to a boil and add the spaghetti. Cook according to the packet instructions. Once cooked, drain and toss with olive oil.

4. Cook the green beans and carrots in a medium pot filled with boiling water for 2-3 minutes.

5. Serve the Bolognese on top of the spaghetti. Sprinkle with cheese and add the vegetables on the side.

Minestrone

Cal 386	**Difficulty:** Easy **Preparation time:** 10 minutes **Cook time:** 40 minutes **Servings:** 4

Nutrition per serving (g)

Fat	Saturates	Carbs	Sugars	Fiber	Protein	Salt
17	3.9	50	11.8	10.6	11.9	1.1

Ingredients

- 3 oz bacon, optional
- 1 cup leeks, green parts
- 2 carrots, large
- 1 small potato
- ¼ cup celery, no more than 2 inches of stalk
- 1 tbsp garlic-infused oil
- 1 tsp olive oil
- 2 cups spinach
- ¾ cup zucchini
- 2 cans (15 oz each) of tomato, crushed
- 2 cups vegetable stock, no garlic or onion
- 1 ¼ cups boiling water
- ½ cup basil, fresh
- ½ cup gluten-free pasta, spirals or shells
- 1 cup chickpeas, in brine, drained
- 2 tbsp Parmesan, optional

Method

1. Dice the potato and carrots. Slice the celery and leeks. Remove the rind off the bacon before dicing. Add the garlic-infused oil, carrots, bacon, potatoes, celery, and leeks to a pan and sauté over medium heat for 15-20 minutes. These vegetables should be soft but not brown.

2. Dice the zucchini and slice the spinach. Make the stock by following the instructions on the packaging. Drain and rinse the chickpeas.

3. Add the tomatoes, stock, hot water, zucchini, spinach, and chickpeas to the pot. Summer for 10 minutes over medium heat.

4. Add the pasta and basil to the soup, setting aside a little basil for a garnish. Cook the pasta according to the instructions on the packet, using the soup as the water.

5. Season and garnish with basil and Parmesan.

Vegetable Fried Rice

Cal 310

Difficulty: Easy
Preparation time: 5 minutes
Cook time: 15 minutes
Servings: 2

Nutrition per serving (g)

Fat	Saturates	Carbs	Sugars	Fiber	Protein	Salt
17.1	5.8	28.2	4.3	2.1	10.7	0.5

Ingredients

- 1 ½ cups rice, cooked and cooled
- 1 ½ tsp garlic-infused oil
- 2 eggs, whisked
- 2 carrots, chopped finely
- 2 cups vegetables (zucchini, bell peppers, and leeks), chopped into cubes
- 4 spring onions, green parts
- Pinch of salt
- 1 tbsp ginger, minced
- 2 tbsp sesame oil
- 1 tbsp soy sauce
- 1 tsp chili flakes, crushed

Method

1. In a large pan over medium heat, heat 1 tablespoon of garlic-infused oil. Add the egg, and cook until scrambled, stirring occasionally. Transfer the egg to another plate.

2. Heat the remaining ½ teaspoon of oil over medium heat, then add the carrots and other vegetables. Cook for 8 minutes until the carrot is soft.

3. Add the rice, onion, ginger, salt, and soy sauce to the pan. Stir for 3 minutes, then mix the egg into the dish.

4. Remove from the heat and stir in the sesame oil and chili flakes before serving.

Roasted Pumpkin and Carrot Soup

Cal: 245 — VEGAN

Difficulty: Medium
Preparation time: 15 minutes
Cook time: 55 minutes
Servings: 6

Nutrition per serving (g)

Fat	Saturates	Carbs	Sugars	Fiber	Protein	Salt
13.6	2.4	27	15.8	9	5.6	0.3

Ingredients

- 7 cups pumpkin, peeled and cubed
- 4 ½ cups carrots, peeled and cubed
- 3 tbsp olive oil
- 1 ½ tbsp garlic-infused oil
- 2 tsp coriander, ground
- 1 tsp cumin, ground
- 1 tsp turmeric, ground
- ½ tsp cardamom, ground
- ¼ tsp chili powder
- 4 ½ cups vegetable stock, no onion or garlic
- 2 ¼ cups water

Method

1. Preheat the oven to 400°F. On a lined tray, place the carrots and pumpkin and drizzle with oil. Bake for 35 minutes.

2. Heat the remainder of the oil in a pot, then add the seeds and spices. Allow them to cook until the mustard seeds pop.

3. Place all the ingredients into the pot and cook for 15 minutes.

4. Allow the mixture to cool for 15 minutes and then blend and serve.

Feta Meatball

Cal 619

Difficulty: Easy
Preparation time: 15 minutes
Cook time: 15 minutes
Servings: 1

Nutrition per serving (g)

Fat	Saturates	Carbs	Sugars	Fiber	Protein	Salt
44	12.5	9	2.7	2.9	44	0.3

Ingredients

- 1 lb lean ground beef
- ⅓ cup feta cheese
- 2 slices bread, crumbled
- 2 ½ tbsp parsley, chopped
- 1 ½ tbsp tomato paste
- 1 cup cherry tomatoes
- 1 lb pasta
- A drizzle of red wine vinegar
- ¼ cup kale, chopped
- 1 tbsp basil, firmly packed
- 2 tbsp roasted almonds
- 1 ½ tbsp garlic-infused oil
- 4 tbsp olive oil
- 2 ½ tbsp lemon juice
- 1 tbsp Parmesan cheese

Method

1. Preheat the oven to 425° F and line a baking tray with parchment paper.

2. First, make the pesto. Place the kale, basil, Parmesan, and almonds into a food processor and mix until finely chopped. Slowly add the oil and lemon in a thin stream. Once mixed, set aside.

3. In a bowl, mix the ground beef, feta, bread crumbs, tomato paste, and parsley. Once mixed together, roll the mixture into balls. Use about a tablespoon of mixture per ball. After rolling, place them onto the baking tray. Drizzle with a small amount of olive oil and bake for 10 minutes. Add the tomatoes and bake for 10 more minutes.

4. While the meatballs are in the oven, cook the pasta according to the instructions on the package. When draining, keep ⅓ of the pasta water. Add the pesto and pasta water to the pot with the pasta.

5. Serve with the meatballs, tomatoes, and a small amount of red wine vinegar.

Spicy Tacos

Cal 450

Difficulty: Easy
Preparation time: 20 minutes
Cook time: 10 minutes
Servings: 6

Nutrition per serving (g)

Fat	Saturates	Carbs	Sugars	Fiber	Protein	Salt
27	12	17	2.5	5	33	0.3

Ingredients

Seasoning

- 2 ½ tsp ground cumin
- 1 ½ tsp smoked paprika
- 1 tsp chili powder
- 1 tsp dried oregano
- ½ tsp black pepper

Filling

- 1 lb your choice of protein (chicken, fish, or ground beef)
- 2 tomatoes, diced
- 2 lettuce leaves, large
- 1 jalapeño
- 12 corn tortillas
- 1 cup shredded cheddar cheese
- 1 cup coriander, fresh and chopped
- Thick Greek yogurt

Method

1. Mix the seasoning ingredients together in a jar or bowl.

2. In a heated pan greased with oil, add the seasoning and stir for 30 seconds. Then, add the protein and cook thoroughly.

3. Fill the tortillas with the vegetables and protein. Top with coriander and yogurt and serve.

Gnocchi

Cal 504	Difficulty: Medium Preparation time: 5 minutes Cook time: 20 minutes Servings: 2

Nutrition per serving (g)

Fat	Saturates	Carbs	Sugars	Fiber	Protein	Salt
19	3.8	65.9	4.5	4.9	13.5	0.3

Ingredients

- 2 tbsp blanched almonds, toasted and chopped
- 1 tbsp garlic-infused oil
- 2 tbsp olive oil
- 2 tbsp Parmesan
- ½ cup cherry tomatoes, cut in half
- ¼ cup green beans
- 1 lb gnocchi
- 1 lemon, juiced
- ¼ cup rocket
- Pepper to taste
- Salt to taste
- 1 tbsp olive oil

Method

1. In a pot, combine a pinch of salt and water, filling half the pot, and boil over high heat.

2. In a small bowl, add the almonds and a pinch of salt and pepper.

3. Mix the finely chopped basil with 1 tablespoon olive oil and 1 tablespoon garlic. Add to the bowl with the almonds and salt. Grate half the Parmesan into the bowl with salt and pepper.

4. Add the halved tomatoes to the mix, and use your hands to mix everything together.

5. Trim and boil the green beans in a small pot for 4 minutes. Once tender, cut into strips lengthwise.

Vegan Curry

Cal 471 VEGAN

Difficulty: Easy
Preparation time: 20 minutes
Cook time: 40 minutes
Servings: 4

Nutrition per serving (g)

Fat	Saturates	Carbs	Sugars	Fiber	Protein	Salt
29	11.9	38.9	12	8	8.4	0.5

Ingredients

- 1 ½ cups pumpkin or sweet potato
- 1 cup carrots
- 1 cup eggplant
- ½ bunch fresh coriander
- 1 cup canned chickpeas in water, rinsed
- 1 ½ tbsp olive oil
- ¼ tsp chili flakes
- 1 ½ tsp ground coriander
- 1 tsp ground turmeric
- 1 tsp ground cumin
- 2 tsp crushed ginger
- 2 tbsp garlic-infused oil
- ½ cup green tips of spring onions
- ½ cup coconut milk, canned
- 1 cup vegetable stock, no onion or garlic
- 1 dried bay leaf
- 1 ½ tbsp soy sauce
- 2 ½ tbsp tomato paste
- 1 lime, zest
- 1 tsp sugar
- 1 ½ cups cooked basmati rice
- 2 tbsp cornstarch

Method

1. Preheat the oven to 350°F. Place the chickpeas and eggplant on a lined tray. Cook for 10 minutes, then flip the eggplant and chickpeas and cook for another 10 minutes.

2. While the eggplant and chickpeas are in the oven, cook the rice according to the instructions on the packet.

3. In a large frying pan over medium heat, add the spices, garlic oil, and spring onion. Fry for two minutes.

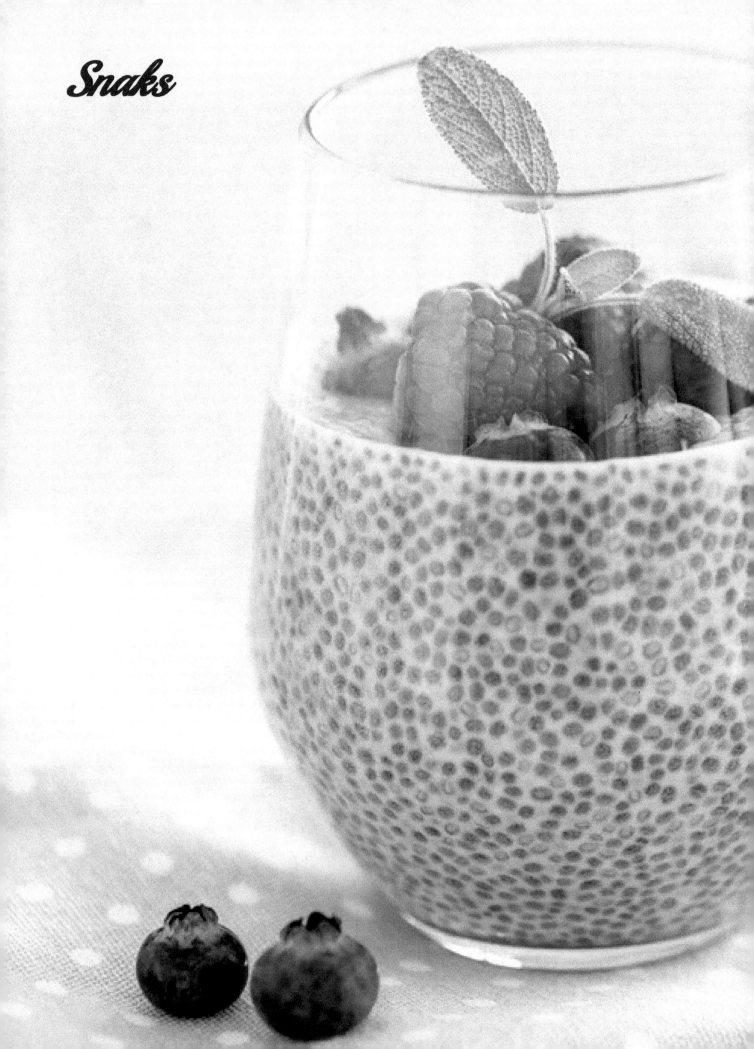

Snaks

Quinoa Muffins

Cal 175

Difficulty: Easy
Preparation time: 10 minutes
Cook time: 20 minutes
Servings: 24 muffins (1 per serving)

Nutrition per serving (g)

Fat	Saturates	Carbs	Sugars	Fiber	Protein	Salt
10.5	4	6	4	1.5	14	0.5

Ingredients

- 1 ½ cups quinoa flour
- 1 cup quinoa flakes
- ⅓ cup walnuts, chopped
- 1 tbsp cinnamon
- 4 tsp baking powder
- 2 tsp baking soda
- Pinch of salt
- 4 eggs
- 4 bananas, mashed
- ½ cup almond milk
- ¼ cup maple syrup

Method

1. Preheat the oven to 375°F.

2. Mix the dry ingredients in one bowl. In a separate bowl, combine the wet ingredients. Combine the ingredients until mixed fully.

3. Spoon into greased muffin pans and bake for 20 minutes. Check if the center is dry by poking the center of a muffin with a skewer. If it comes out clean, they are ready.

Chocolate Peanut Butter Energy Bites

Cal 240
VEGAN

Difficulty: Easy
Preparation time: 10 minutes
Cook time: 2 minutes
Servings: 10 (2 bites per serving)

Nutrition per serving (g)

Fat	Saturates	Carbs	Sugars	Fiber	Protein	Salt
11	1	29	9	4	8	0.6

Ingredients

- ½ cup smooth peanut butter
- 1 cup oats
- ⅓ cup maple syrup
- ¼ cup peanuts, roasted, chopped
- ¼ cup dark chocolate, 55%, finely chopped
- Pinch of salt

Method

1. In a bowl, mix the ingredients.

2. Once mixed, roll the mixture into balls (approximately 1 tablespoon in size, add more if there is mixture left once 10 balls have been rolled). They will need to be compressed as they are rolled. Store in an airtight container.

Summer Popsicle

Cal 156 — VEGAN

Difficulty: Easy
Preparation time: 15 minutes
Cook time: 2 minutes
Servings: 4 (5 ½ tbsp per popsicle)

Nutrition per serving (g)

Fat	Saturates	Carbs	Sugars	Fiber	Protein	Salt
0.5	0.1	38.9	19.2	9.7	2.7	0.1

Ingredients

- 4 carrots, large
- 3 oranges, large
- 1 lime, juiced
- 1 tsp orange zest
- 2 tbsp powdered sugar

Method

1. Grate the carrots.

2. In a clean cloth, wrap the carrots and squeeze the juice into a bowl.

3. Zest an orange. Juice the oranges and lime into the bowl of carrot juice and mix the zest in. Add the powdered sugar. If the mixture tastes too sour, add more powdered sugar, then pour into popsicle molds.

4. Place in the freezer overnight. If using wooden sticks, place them in after 2 hours in the freezer.

Orange Biscuits

Cal 154

Difficulty: Easy
Preparation time: 25 minutes
Cook time: 25 minutes
Servings: 24 (1-2 per serving)

Nutrition per serving (g)

Fat	Saturates	Carbs	Sugars	Fiber	Protein	Salt
4.1	0.6	27.8	14.6	1.7	1.3	0.1

Ingredients

Biscuits

- ½ tsp of baking soda
- Pinch of salt
- 2 cups flour, gluten-free or oat
- 1 tsp orange zest
- ½ cup butter
- ½ cup brown sugar
- ½ cup white sugar
- 1 egg, large
- 2 tbsp orange juice, fresh
- 1 tsp vanilla extract

Glaze

- 1 cup powdered sugar
- 1 ½ tsp orange zest
- 1 ½ tbsp orange juice, fresh

Method

1. Preheat the oven to 350°F.

2. Use a grater to zest the orange. Do not grate the white layer.

3. Whisk the salt, baking soda, zest, and flour together in a large bowl.

4. In a different bowl, beat the butter and sugar together using an electric hand beater until the mixture is fluffy and not grainy. Add 2 tablespoons of orange juice, the egg, and the vanilla to the mixture.

5. Combine the dry and wet ingredients and mix until the dough is sticky. Form balls using about 2 tablespoons of dough. Place the balls on trays that are covered in parchment paper, then flatten the dough slightly before baking for 15-20 minutes. Rotate the trays halfway through. When the edges are golden brown, remove the trays and let them cool down on cooling racks.

6. For the icing, mix the powdered sugar, orange juice, and zest together. The icing should be sticky and not runny. Use a teaspoon to ice the biscuits once they are cool.

Coconut Bites

Cal 139	**Difficulty:** Easy **Preparation time:** 15 minutes **Cook time:** 2 minutes **Servings:** 14 (4 bites per serving)

Nutrition per serving (g)

Fat	Saturates	Carbs	Sugars	Fiber	Protein	Salt
8,2	2.5	14.9	8	0.8	1.8	0.1

Ingredients

- 2 cups cornflakes, gluten-free
- ½ cup brown sugar
- ¼ cup oats
- 6 tbsp dried coconut, shredded
- 4 tbsp pumpkin seeds
- 6 tbsp butter

Method

1. Crush the cornflakes and soften the butter. Place all the ingredients, except the coconut, into a food processor and pulse until large crumbs form.

2. Press and roll the mixture into balls, approximately 1 tbsp per ball (add more if there is leftover dough), then roll in the coconut.

3. Store in the fridge.

Energy Bars

Cal 121	Difficulty: Easy Preparation time: 10 minutes Cook time: - Servings: 14 (1 slice per serving)

Nutrition per serving (g)						
Fat	Saturates	Carbs	Sugars	Fiber	Protein	Salt
6.4	1	14.4	8.8	1.2	3	0

Ingredients

- ⅓ cup sunflower seed butter or peanut butter
- 6 tbsp maple syrup
- 1 ½ cups puffed rice
- ½ cup pumpkin seeds, roughly chopped
- 4 tbsp dried cranberries, chopped roughly
- ½ tsp ginger, ground
- ½ tsp cinnamon, ground
- 1 tbsp dark chocolate, chopped roughly

Method

1. Line a square baking pan with parchment paper.

2. Melt the butter and the syrup over medium heat. Once melted, remove from the heat and stir in the pumpkin seeds, puffed rice, dried cranberries, ginger, and cinnamon. Coat the ingredients evenly.

3. Spread the mixture across the pan evenly, then place another piece of parchment paper over the mixture and apply pressure evenly to compress.

4. Melt the dark chocolate, then drizzle over the mixture. Refrigerate for 2 hours before cutting

Conclusion

It is true that most people who live with diverticulosis may never develop diverticulitis (which is the inflammation of any of the pouches on the lining of the colon). Still, about 200,000 people in America suffer the uncomfortable symptoms of diverticulitis every year.

As such, there is the need for a book that illuminates this subject and provides adequate solutions. Hopefully, **Diverticulitis Cookbook** has been useful to you in this regard.

Others books by Robert Dickens

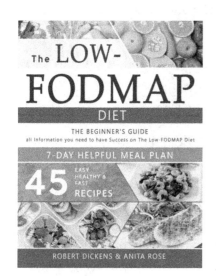

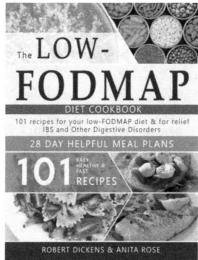

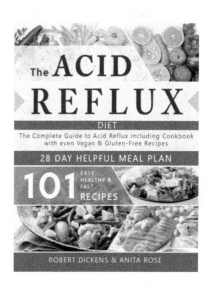

The Low-FODMAP diet

The Beginner's Guide, including 7 days Meal Plan + 45 Easy, healthy & fast recipes and all information you need to have Success on The Low-FODMAP Diet

Low FODMAP diet cookbook

101 Easy, healthy & fast recipes for yours low-FODMAP diet + 28 days helpful meal plans

The Acid Reflux Diet

The Complete Guide to heal your Acid Reflux & GERD + 28 days healpfull meal plans Including Cookbook with 101 recipes even Vegan & Gluten-Free recipes

References

A guide to the low-FODMAP diet for reducing IBS symptoms. (2020). Gutcare. https://www.gutcare.com.sg/a-guide-to-the-low-fodmap-diet-for-reducing-ibs-symptoms/

Coble, L. J., Sheldon, E. K., Yue, F., Salameh, J. T., Harris, R. L., Deiling, S., Ruggiero, M. F., Eshelman, A. M., et al. (2017). Identification of a rare LAMB4 variant associated with familial diverticulitis through exome sequencing. Human Molecular Genetics, 26(16), 3212-3220. https://doi.org/10.1093/hmg/ddx204

Coppola, S. (2020). Foods to avoid if you have diverticulitis. Healthline. https://www.healthline.com/health/diverticulitis-diet-list-of-foods-to-avoid#:~:text=It%20stands%20for%20fermentable%20oligosaccharides,that%20are%20high%20in%20FODMAPS.

Drossman, A. D., Morris, B. C., Schneck, S., Hu, J. Y., Norton, J. N., Norton, F. W., Weinland, S., Dalton, C., et al. (2010). International survey of people with IBS. Journal of Clinical Gastroenterology, 43(6), 541-550. https://doi.org/10.1097/MCG.0b013e318189a7f9

Persons, L. (2019). Everything you need to know about diverticulitis. Healthline. https://www.healthline.com/health/diverticulitis#diverticulitis-vs.-diverticulosis

Stollman, N., Smalley, W., & Ikuo, H. (2015). American Gastroenterological Association Institute Guideline on the management of acute diverticulitis. Gastroenterology, 149(7), 1944-1949. https://doi.org/10.1053/j.gastro.2015.10.003

© **Copyright 2021 - All rights reserved.**

The content contained within this book may not be reproduced, duplicated or transmitted without direct written permission from the author or the publisher.

Under no circumstances will any blame or legal responsibility be held against the publisher, or author, for any damages, reparation, or monetary loss due to the information contained within this book, either directly or indirectly.

Legal Notice:
This book is copyright protected. It is only for personal use. You cannot amend, distribute, sell, use, quote or paraphrase any part, or the content within this book, without the consent of the author or publisher.

Disclaimer Notice:
Please note the information contained within this document is for educational and entertainment purposes only. All effort has been executed to present accurate, up to date, reliable, complete information. No warranties of any kind are declared or implied. Readers acknowledge that the author is not engaged in the rendering of legal, financial, medical or professional advice. The content within this book has been derived from various sources. Please consult a licensed professional before attempting any techniques outlined in this book.

By reading this document, the reader agrees that under no circumstances is the author responsible for any losses, direct or indirect, that are incurred as a result of the use of the information contained within this document, including, but not limited to, errors, omissions, or inaccuracies.

CPSIA information can be obtained
at www.ICGtesting.com
Printed in the USA
LVHW100755250421
685460LV00003B/51